1935 1985

THE HAMMERSMITH

THE FIRST FIFTY YEARS

1935 1985

THE HAMMERSMITH

THE FIRST FIFTY YEARS

of the
Royal Postgraduate Medical School
at
Hammersmith Hospital

by James Calnan FRCS FRCP

Emeritus Professor of Plastic and Reconstructive Surgery
in the University of London at the Royal Postgraduate Medical School,
Honorary Consultant Surgeon, Hammersmith Hospital

MTP PRESS LIMITED
a member of the KLUWER ACADEMIC PUBLISHERS GROUP
LANCASTER / BOSTON / THE HAGUE / DORDRECHT

Published in the UK and Europe by
MTP Press Limited,
Falcon House,
Lancaster, England

British Library Cataloguing in Publication Data

Calnan, James
The Hammersmith 1935–1985: the first 50 years
of the Royal Postgraduate Medical School at
Hammersmith hospital.
1. Royal Postgraduate Medical School—History
I. Title
610'.7'1142133 R773.R6/

ISBN-13:978-94-011-6360-6 e-ISBN-13:978-94-011-6358-3

DOI: 10.1007/978-94-011-6358-3

Published in the USA by MTP Press
a division of Kluwer Boston Inc
190 Old Derby Street,
Hingham,
MA 02043, USA

Library of Congress Cataloging in Publication Data

Calnan, James.
The Hammersmith, 1935–1985.

Bibliography: p.
Includes index.
1. Royal Postgraduate Medical School—History.
2. Medical—Study and teaching (Continuing education)—
England—London—History. 3. Hammersmith Hospital—
History. I. Hammersmith Hospital. II. Royal
Postgraduate Medical School. III. Title. [DNLM:
1. Schools, Medical—history—London. 2. Education,
Medical, Continuing—history—London. W 20 C164h]
R845.C35 1985 610'.7'1142133 85-5216

Filmset by Vantage Photosetting Co Ltd
Eastleigh and London

Contents

Acknowledgements

I gratefully acknowledge assistance in preparing this book from the following:

1. The Wellcome Trust for a generous donation towards the cost of producing the many photographs.
2. Dr J. Welsman Ph.D., School Secretary, and Dr W. F. Bynum M.D., Ph.D., Head of the Academic Unit, Wellcome Institute for the History of Medicine, both of whom read drafts and made valuable comments.
3. Mr Doig Simmonds Aol, A.M.A., Head of the Department of Medical Illustration at the school, for the cover design and help with the layout.
4. Mr David Hawtin B.A. (Hons), Chief Photographer, who produced the photographs which illustrate, as much as the script, what the school was and is.
5. Professors David Hill and Donald Moss, archivists, for permission to use material collected by them.
6. The many friends and colleagues who talked to me, gave of their time and may not have been mentioned in the book.

James Calnan

1

Explanations and Definitions

Anyone coming on site today would be confused by the presence of Hammersmith Hospital administered by a Special Health Authority of the National Health Service, the Royal Postgraduate Medical School – an independent School within the University of London – and various autonomous units of the Medical Research Council. Each has its own staff, administration, organization, financial arrangements and work practices, yet all manage to live amicably alongside. Probably if the general public was asked, most would have heard of Hammersmith Hospital, few of the Royal Postgraduate Medical School (R.P.M.S.), fewer still of the Medical Research Council (M.R.C.).

Yet the R.P.M.S. at Hammersmith Hospital holds a special place as a pioneer academic institution of postgraduate teaching in London. It is a leading international centre for clinical teaching and research, incorporated by Royal Charter in 1931, and was opened as a School of the University of London on 13 May 1935 by King George V. In 1947 the School became part of the newly formed British Postgraduate Medical Federation, but reverted to independence in 1974. It has 13 academic departments in several buildings on the Hammersmith Hospital site, a paid and honorary staff of 180 – including 24 Professors and 9 Readers – making the total number of employees about 740.

Since 1935 more than 25,000 postgraduates drawn from all parts of the world have been registered. Centred as it is on a general hospital, the School has been able to integrate a wide range of specialties, with clinical studies being firmly founded in the basic sciences through strong paraclinical departments. To these 25,000 world-wide, the site is known as 'The Hammersmith', and with the passing of years it will become more difficult to separate School from Hospital or M.R.C.; the view expressed in 1935, and still today, that 'postgraduate medical education must be rooted in the laboratory and the ward' makes any attempt at separation foolish. The original organization of the Hammersmith, unique in the United Kingdom, has survived to this day. The majority of the full-time senior medical staff of the Hospital – the consultants – are still provided not by the National Health Service, but from the senior academic staff of the School. They are Professors, Readers and Senior Lecturers of the University of London, of which the Royal Postgraduate Medical School is a part. This arrangement has facilitated the rapid cross-fertilization of ideas between the laboratory and the ward, and the prompt introduction of scientific discoveries for the treatment of patients. Moreover, as an exclusively postgraduate school unconstrained by the staffing requirements for teaching an undergraduate curriculum, the Hammersmith possessed the flexibility to redistribute resources from one area of activity to another in order to support new, exciting and innovative ideas.

Today over 1500 students each year receive postgraduate education in 13 academic departments of the School, some for periods as short as 1 week, others as part of courses that may last 3 years. In 1948 the School prospectus referred to only one diploma course, that of the D.C.P., which started in 1935. In the 1984 prospectus there were four Master's degree courses (the M.Sc. in Experimental Pathology (Toxicology), Medical Microbiology, Clinical Biochemistry, Nuclear Medicine) and five diploma courses (in Clinical Pathology, Applied Medical Research (Endocrinology), Haematology, Immunology, and Cardiology) besides the training in research leading to the degrees of Master of Philosophy (M.Phil.) and Doctor of Philosophy (Ph.D.); M.D. and M.S. theses are commonplace. Although the library holds copies of only 304 theses, almost entirely Ph.D.s sent on from the university senate and locked away in the basement for reasons of copyright, this total is far short of those successful in the past 50 years. At any given time 50% of the student body is likely to come from 70 different countries overseas, and the School would be a very different and intellectually poorer institution without them.

Whilst the courses and research organized by the staff of the School cover a wide area, one feature common to all of them is that they are carried out by the same full-time academic staff who direct the clinical practice of Hammersmith Hospital, an arrangement that is unique in the U.K. and arises from the '1951 Agreement'. Hammersmith Hospital is, therefore, a teaching hospital in a very special sense, even in London.

The three principles embodied in the Royal Charter of 1931 – that:

- the School would concentrate entirely on postgraduate education (especially for those who came from overseas) and no undergraduates would be admitted,

- the educational programme would be directed by full-time academic staff,
- the work of the School would cover all the major clinical and paraclinical disciplines in its approach –

have been preserved during the past 50 years; they have shaped the structure of the School and have determined its ethos ever since. These composite principles have been demonstrated as a valuable and successful way of promoting effective postgraduate medical education. The figures of past successes confirm this ethos and there seems no valid reason to discard it.

THE HAMMERSMITH ETHOS

The Greek word 'ethos', meaning 'character', and inferring the ideal of excellence, has come to define an attitude of mind, a way of life, essentially abstract, but which can be recognized by practical acts. In the last 50 years there has developed at Hammersmith a certain attitude to medicine that others recognize as the Hammersmith ethos, difficult to define but worth the attempt.

First, because everyone on site is involved in research of one kind or another – usually for self-recognition, career advancement, genuine curiosity, excitement and sheer fun, all mixed together – people are watchful and opportunist so that the basic attitude of 'observation' is ever present in clinical practice, casual conversation, scientific meetings, and everyday reading. Indeed a daily visit to the library becomes as natural as toiletry. The aims of those who come to the Hammersmith are clear before they arrive; they know why they come, for achievement. The incentives of publications of career advancement – even a personal chair – maintain the original driving force.

Second, the concern with original ideas, almost irrespective of whether they are useful or important in daily practice, soon becomes part of the personality of those who stay for any length of time, which is not to say that they believe in realism as a matter of faith, however pragmatic their actions.

Third, a certain independence of mind in the attitude to others working in the same field of research or clinical practice – the two are so intimately bound together that it is often difficult to distinguish between them, which is not lost on those who disagree with either – is more difficult to define but was summed up by the reviewer of one of the many successful textbooks published by staff: 'It is not so much that doctors at Hammersmith do things differently, rather that they are indifferent to the ways of others.'

Fourth, that the number of publications from an individual or a department is a good index of performance in research is often denied but secretly admitted. Indeed, a lack of publications is commonly the strongest argument used to deny a colleague access to precious equipment, buildings, or funds.

Moreover there is tacit acknowledgement that the best work is published in the best journals, so that the quality of the research tends to be assessed by the reputation of the journal in which it appears. For instance, in 1980, of the total 620 School and Hospital publications 60% appeared in the best three journals of 15 different specialties.

Fifth, teaching has almost always been by example rather than by formal and didactic methods, which has led to adverse comment by other schools and other universities. The premise that only by continuous research can teaching be true and up to date is not generally accepted elsewhere. Indeed, Medicine is one of the few professions where continuous updating of knowledge is demanded from within the profession.

The courses and seminars put on at the Hammersmith are rarely 'refresher courses' in the generally accepted sense because they contain such a high proportion of new, untried and often unpublished work presented for criticism by the audience. Critical examination in public of data collected with obvious devotion frequently leads to new thoughts, as well as first-class intellectual entertainment. The acceptance of criticism – a word incidentally, which implies condemnation to a politician but which is central to scientific method and to the advancement of knowledge – has stimulated a high proportion of staff to travel and lecture in many parts of the world. In the sixties, B.T.A. (been to America, meaning the U.S.A. and Canada) was almost a required diploma at the School because at that time the U.S.A. was the one country where the Flexner doctrine (of academic units in all major specialties) was extant and so could provide a contest of ideas at staff rounds and scientific meetings. This fervour of international evangelism continues to bring benefits to the Hammersmith in various ways: new ideas and practices are imported, bright young men are encouraged to come and work here, senior colleagues are invited to visit – which at least prevents parochialism, and is an important public relations exercise in its own right; at the same time the research and clinical practices of Hammersmith are exported and subjected to public and private criticism.

This philosophy of medicine, described here as the Hammersmith ethos, has replicated world-wide, irrespective of national cultures, and with minor modifications is just as easily recognizable in the East as in the West. Its origins can be discovered in this book.

The Golden Jubilee of the Hammersmith will be celebrated in 1985. The event should be commemorated by a book detailing the history of those 50 years of endeavour and attainment, but Hammersmith has always been more interested in the future than the past and as a result has been diffident in preserving such items that a historian will need to produce a definitive history. Indeed, it was only in 1977 that Professor David Hill was asked to act as archivist for the Royal Postgraduate Medical School. He did an excellent job, but even so the amount of material salvaged, compared to what could have been preserved, is pitifully small.

ABOUT THIS ACCOUNT

Many past and present staff have advocated that a history should be written, but no one has so far done so – understandably, and for two reasons. First, there is the problem of historical perspective; second the fear that the writing would be anecdotal at best and libellous at worst. My account is a personal view, not a definitive history, for it lacks the perspective of time; but the theme is too important to leave until a more objective assessment can be made. I hope that at some future date the history of the Hammersmith of the past 50 turbulent years will be written with greater detachment, but the lessons of the past half-century are needed today. Survival is a continuing problem as much as discovery. The political threat to elitism and meritocracy in medicine is no less real than the threat to all private enterprise and initiative: yet we need all of these. Hammersmith has withstood the fashionable rejection: of competition, of academic excellence, of personal sacrifice, of faith in the future. Its resilience was built at the time of founding and has been renewed since, but the story needs to be told.

This book differs from others about hospitals and medical schools in at least two respects. It spans a short period of time, just half a century, and it comprises the lifetime of the author and many of his readers. The first makes it possible to go into more detail than usual and to put this in the context of world or national events. The second makes it unusually difficult to see the whole sequence of events and the effects in due perspective and proportions, although the immediacy of interest and atmosphere helps to supplement the effort of interpreting the past.

This book is not a history. I am no historian and do not attempt to produce a scholarly, detailed work – which if dull would be a great injustice to the people and the place – but rather have tried to tell the fascinating story of a group of men and women working in an unusual set of buildings during a time of major changes: in education, research, finance, in national and local social awareness, and in medical advances previously undreamed of. It is the story of an institution that is at once exciting, stimulating, frustrating, yet eminently satisfying; a story that does aim to be readable, accurate, and explanatory.

Readability to a large extent depends on the reader. Hence this book is for those who have been to the Hammersmith, that they may reminisce; for those who are at the Hammersmith, that they may be enlightened by past events and come to understand the reasons for present staffing, buildings, research and clinical practices; for those who might visit in the future so that they are prepared and can interpret more readily what they see and hear, and to know of its strange beginnings and past achievements. And accuracy? I have relied largely on documents and personal observations. For instance when David Hill was consulted about the date of the Golden Jubilee he was able to provide four possibilities: 1981, because the Royal Charter was granted to the School in 1931 and the Governing Body constituted; 1983, because the foundation stone was laid in 1933; 1984, because the first professors were appointed in 1934, the School Council came into existence, and Hammersmith became a recognized School of the University of London; 1985, because the school buildings were occupied in January 1935, probably by piecemeal occupation, and were declared open by King George V on 13 May 1935. So accuracy, too, needs qualification; and because this story concerns people, often in groups, who considered problems although the solution was attributed to one alone, credit must have its own degree of 'tolerance', to use an engineering term, to the reader. With the passage of time such 'inaccuracies' will be sorted out even if the truth remains equivocal. Much of what is thought about as progress is often nothing but change, and some of the Hammersmith story is mainly about change: every story is indeed the projection of the man who writes it and of the culture upon which he draws. If the reader finds this account enjoyable, I am satisfied; if he finds it interesting and accurate by his own knowledge, I am more than pleased.

2

Postgraduate Medical Education: the Problem and a Solution

Lloyd George's National Insurance Act of 1911 had far-reaching consequences besides the well-recognized health scheme and compensation for injured workers. The Medical Research Committee was set up in 1913 as a direct result, to lead and define research, and acquitted itself well during the Great War of 1914–1918. Long before the end of the war Lloyd George had decided that all the provisions of the Act should be implemented as part of the grand design – to create 'a country fit for heroes to live in' – and in 1916 instituted the new Ministry of Reconstruction. Dr Christopher Addison,[1] Member of Parliament for Hoxton in the East End of London and Professor of Anatomy at University College, Sheffield, was to be the first Minister. The choice could hardly have been bettered for he sired a range of committees including one of the machinery of government chaired by Lord Haldane.

For medicine Addison did three things. First, he arranged for the Medical Research Committee to receive a Royal Charter in 1921 and to be formally constituted as the Medical Research Council. For the next 60 years it was to be the premier instrument of medical research; fostering the good, condemning the bad and setting standards that attained world-wide approval.

Second, he created the Ministry of Health in 1919, with Addison as the first Minister, Sir Robert Morant as Permanent Secretary, Sir George Newman (then Chief Medical Officer at the Board of Education and later to be a key figure in the founding of the School) as Chief Medical Officer of Health – 'an extremely far-sighted and resolute group, seeking long-term objectives'.[2] Morant died suddenly in 1920 and Addison, who had become famous for his housing policy of allowing local authorities to build unlimited numbers of council houses after the war, was criticized for their cost and resigned from the Government as a matter of principle. Newman remained, to establish the rights and duties of doctors working as civil servants of the state (their status, pay, right of direct access to the Minister to put forward proposals and to discuss any matter within their responsibility – all of which remain virtually unchanged to this day). One of his memos is particularly pertinent: 'A medical man in the Civil Service has a duty to his profession as well as to the Service, and he should not enter it unless he is prepared to obey orders and work co-operatively and harmoniously in a great organisation.' Newman's principles were extremely flexible and allowed great scope for personal interpretation: regrettably the spirit today, the dead hand of bureaucracy, is to kill initiative, to resent responsibility as evidence of unwarranted power and to make individuals accountable for every minor action.

Third, Addison tackled the permanent problem of postgraduate medical education by setting up a committee of enquiry[3] with Lord Athlone as chairman on 26 January 1921: 'to investigate the needs of medical practitioners and other graduates for further eduction in medicine in London, and to submit proposals for a practical scheme for meeting them' (a commendably brief definition of what was needed).

PREVIOUS POSTGRADUATE EDUCATION

There had been previous attempts to develop postgraduate education and training for doctors, but all had failed to flourish. For instance, Sir Jonathan Hutchinson,[4] Consultant Surgeon to the London Hospital and Professor of Surgery in the University and a Fellow of the Royal Society, who had been President of the Royal College of Surgeons in 1890 and President of the Royal Society of Medicine in 1894, probably saw more than anyone the dire need for postgraduate education and had put on a series of demonstrations at his clinical museum in Great Portland Street. In 1899 with Sir William Broadbent, Physician Extraordinary to Queen Victoria and Consultant Physician at St Mary's Hospital, and with Dr Theodore Williams, Hutchinson (then 71 years old) set up the Medical Graduates' College and Polyclinic in Chenies Street. Daily clinical demonstrations and lectures were given, attended by London doctors, but no hospital was included in the venture. The West London Post-Graduate College was started at the West London Hospital, Hammersmith, in 1893 to provide ward teaching, lectures, daily clinical demonstrations, and instruction in public health. The North-East London Post-Graduate College was opened in 1902 at the Prince of Wales Hospital, Tottenham, and the London School of Clinical Medicine at the Seamen's Hospital, Greenwich, in 1906. All these colleges had links with local hospitals and charged comparable fees of about 3 guineas for 1 month's attendance. With the advent of the Great War all disbanded. In 1918 Sir William Osler founded the Fellowship of

Medicine and Post-Graduate Medical Association. For a fee of 6 guineas the doctor could attend any of the courses of instruction, arranged at a number of general and special hospitals in London, for 1 month; in the following 3 years over 1000 postgraduates were registered, mainly those demobilized before returning to general practice.

All these organizations were successful for a time, but they failed to advance postgraduate medicine, probably because they were all teaching the medicine of the past and not the medicine for the next generation. The real need was for what Starling, the greatest British physiologist of his time, called 'academic medicine'. His oft-quoted words to the Haldane Commission of 1918 were: 'This is what I regard as the University spirit, not diagnosing a patient and deciding what we do for him in order to earn our fee, but what we can get out of this case in order to do better next time. How can we get some knowledge out of this patient in order to have more power when we have another man in the same condition?'

Osler too had spoken to the Haldane Commission: 'Just as professors of chemistry need a laboratory and assistants, so a professor of medicine needs a Hospital Unit of beds, laboratories and assistants, to enable him to treat, to teach and to research.' Charles Newman[5] stated that Osler got his ideas from Welch at Johns Hopkins Hospital, who got his from Kohnheim, derived originally from Von Humboldt during the redevelopment of the academic spirit in German universities. Certainly, Haldane greatly admired the German academic system – as did many other learned medical men as late as 1933 who often encouraged students to visit and study in Berlin or Vienna during the long summer vacation – and couched his final report strongly in its favour: the Kaiser's War made this an unpopular view, but at the end of the war Osler took it up again. He said, 'the profession must get over its infantile fears of government finances and must start to think about postgraduate education on an imperial scale'. Few did or could.

Osler founded the Fellowship of Medicine in 1918 with these ideas in mind but unfortunately died in December 1919, and the Fellowship developed along lines different from Osler's. Even in late 1919 Sir Clifford Allbutt, Regius Professor of Physic at Cambridge (and later to give evidence to the Athlone committee of 1921), said: 'All previous attempts at postgraduate education in this country have failed, and must fail, unless they are rooted in the laboratory and the ward.'

THE ATHLONE COMMITTEE OF 1921

Addison's committee of ten members, chaired by the Earl of Athlone, met on 26 occasions at the Ministry of Health in Whitehall, received 70 memoranda from different bodies and persons, and heard oral evidence from 58. The committee included seven doctors (of whom Herringham, Makins, Newman and Perry were knights of the realm) and reported 4 months later, on 31 May 1921, to the new Minister of Health, Sir Alfred Mond. The plan for a great central institute of postgraduate medical education was certainly ambitious. The recommendations were summarized as follows:

1. A School attached to a Hospital centrally situated in London should be devoted solely to post-graduate medical education.
2. The School should be a School of the University of London, and receive substantial financial assistance from the Treasury through the University Grants Committee.
3. In addition to the courses provided at the Central School for full-time instruction of general practitioners, and at existing post-graduate colleges and schools, further facilities for post-graduate study should be made available at non-teaching hospitals and in Poor Law Infirmaries.
4. It is desirable that increased use should be made of cottage hospitals in which all general practitioners of the neighbourhood should have the right, if they so desire, to treat their patients.
5. A much larger number of resident appointments and clinical assistantships should be created in hospitals and Poor Law Infirmaries.
6. A Central Office should be established to co-ordinate and develop the work of post-graduate education in London. In the administrative building should be provided not only offices but the accommodation necessary for social purposes.
7. An Institute of State Medicine should be established by the University of London in which instruction should be given in public health, Forensic Medicine, Industrial Medicine, and in medical ethics and economics.

The Athlone report was accepted, but little happened. Items 3, 4 and 5 were only realized in the immediate post-war years, from about 1946 onwards; item 6 became the Postgraduate Medical Federation in 1947 and item 7 became the School of Hygiene and Tropical Medicine opened by Edward, the Prince of Wales, in 1929 and aided by a generous grant from the Rockefeller Foundation.

THE CHAMBERLAIN COMMITTEE

In July 1925 Neville Chamberlain, then Minister of Health, set up a postgraduate Medical Education Committee,[6] 'To draw up a practicable scheme of medical education centred in London.' Chamberlain chaired the committee of 14 eminent doctors only one of whom, Sir George Newman, Chief Medical Officer to the Ministry of Health, had sat on the Athlone Committee. The committee's 18 recommendations were reported to Parliament 5 years later, in April 1930, by the Minister of Health, Arthur

Greenwood. The report covered much the same ground as had the Athlone Committee: the need for postgraduate education in general and especially in London (the present urgency); but it accepted five important guides for any proposed institution for postgraduate education:

1. Adaptation of premises already built, and not a new building.
2. School and hospital must be adjacent on the same site; the site should be capable of expansion.
3. The hospital should have no less than 400 beds.
4. The School should teach postgraduates only and not admit undergraduates.
5. The institute should be conveniently located in relation to the medical centre of London.

The 12 general hospitals in London,[7] that is the voluntary hospitals with teaching schools attached, promptly declined to become the British Post-Graduate Medical School, on these conditions, although there had been preliminary discussions with them.

The Committee examined other options, particularly the West London Hospital, a voluntary hospital opened in 1856 (of 225 beds but without a medical school) on a 2½ acre site. Detailed discussions took place in March 1927. The Board of Management of the West London was formally invited to plan its expansion to 400 beds even though, as a voluntary hospital, the Board would have to finance the extra beds. On 22 January 1929 the Board of Management of the West London Hospital agreed to establish the British Postgraduate Hospital and Medical School on their site. The Chamberlain committee had second thoughts and when the Local Government Act was ratified by Parliament, unexpectedly quickly on 27 March 1929, the West London plan was abandoned. Instead, two public hospitals due to be taken over by the London County Council on 1 April 1930,[8] out of 30 possible institutions, were inspected: Lewisham and Hammersmith. 'After devoting a considerable period to a close examination and consideration of these two Hospitals, the Committee unanimously selected the Hammersmith Hospital as affording the most suitable basis for comparison of the alternative means of devising a practicable scheme.' It had exactly 400 beds, 'of which 234 are at present assigned to medical and surgical cases generally, 116 to gynaecological and obstetrical cases and 50 to children'. The long hunt for a hospital in London to which to attach a new kind of medical school was over. The report was published on 23 January 1930, and reported to Parliament by Arthur Greenwood (who had become Minister of Health in June 1929) on 9 April 1930. He set up a Provisional Organizing Committee on 2 July 1930 to pursue:

- the action requisite to lead up to the planning and construction of the Medical School, and

- the form of government appropriate to the Hospital and Medical School, with special reference to the position of London County Council as the Local Authority responsible for the Hospital, and to the position of the University of London in relation to the Medical School.

Viscount Chelmsford[9] was to be Chairman, and Heseltine (Assistant Secretary to the Ministry of Health) Secretary of a Committee of 28 others: these included four from the University of London, four from voluntary hospitals, four from the London County Council, nine from individual undergraduate medical schools, and others from the Ministry of Health, the Medical Research Council and the Royal Colleges. This rather large Committee reported in writing to the Minister on 30 March 1931 with the recommendation that 'the Governing Body of the Medical School is constituted at the earliest possible moment'.

The Provisional Organizing Committee had divided into two subcommittees: Constitution and Education. Both reports had appendices, the first a draft charter, the second a great deal of detail about salaries, courses and organization.

THE 1931 ROYAL CHARTER

The Royal Charter was granted by King George V on 10 July 1931 (although actually worded 'in the twenty-second year of Our Reign') 'to secure new and extended education facilities for the further education of medical practitioners, with the objects of promoting the advancement of knowledge of the best methods of treatment of the sick, and the improved application of such methods in Great Britain and Northern Ireland, the British Dominions, Colonies, and Possessions, and in other countries, it is intended to invite Parliament to vote a sum of money for the provision and equipment of a British Postgraduate Medical School (hereinafter called 'the School') in London . . .'. The charter appointed the foundation governors to plan and build the school, appoint staff, arrange management, co-ordinate with other authorities, provide accommodation for postgraduate students, and become part of the university. The governors were to hold office for 3 years initially, but future governors for 1 year only and be appointed by various bodies, including the Royal Colleges; the London County Council; the Secretaries of State for Dominion Affairs, for India, for the Colonies; University of London; and Minister of Health. A School Council was to be established, by the Governing Body, of three physicians, three surgeons, three representatives of the Hospital medical and scientific staff, University Professors of the School and Heads of Departments, the Dean, and the Medical Officer of the London County Council. The function of the School Council was to consider and report on academic matters of education, university appointments, communication with other universities and examining bodies and General Medical Council, and 'the discipline of students admitted to the School'.

The first Governing Body had 14 members, of whom 11 were doctors. The Governors were:

1. Frederick Goodenough[10], Secretary of State for Dominion Affairs.
2. Lieutenant-Colonel Hugh Dutton, Secretary of State for India, and a doctor retired from the Indian Medical Service.
3. Ambrose Stanton, Secretary of State for the Colonies, also a doctor.
4. Viscount Chelmsford, nominated by the Minister of Health.
5. Sir George Newman, Chief Medical Officer to the Ministry of Health.
6. Miss Florence Lambert, Chief Medical Officer of the London County Council.
7. Lewis Silkin, nominated by the London County Council.
8. Herbert Eason, Senior Ophthalmic Surgeon at Guy's Hospital, nominated by the Senate of the University of London.
9. George Gask, Professor of Surgery in the University of London and a member of the Radium Commission.
10. Lord Dawson of Penn, President of the Royal College of Physicians of London and Physician to the London Hospital.
11. Lord Moynihan of Leeds, President of the Royal College of Surgeons of England, Consulting Surgeon to Leeds General Infirmary and Emeritus Professor of Surgery, University of Leeds.
12. Dr Reginald Wall, President of the Society of Apothecaries of London.
13. Dr Thomas Eden, President of the Royal Society of Medicine.
14. Sir Robert Bolam, Honorary Physician, Royal Victoria Hospital, Newcastle-upon-Tyne, and past Chairman of Council, British Medical Association.

There was a great deal to do before the School opened in 1935. The 10-year interval of inertia between the Athlone Report of 1921 and the Charter of 1931 needs some explanation and consideration: that decade had been a time of many political changes and general instability of government, finance, and social attitudes, all of which had interfered to a greater or lesser extent with the progress of postgraduate medical education.

3

Hammersmith Hospital

Until 1903 the sick poor of the parish of Hammersmith had been taken to Fulham Infirmary, which was administered by a Joint Board of Guardians for Fulham and Hammersmith. In that year Hammersmith Borough was given a separate Board who undertook to build their own infirmary. The site chosen was next to H.M. Prison, Wormwood Scrubs, in Du Cane Road. The foundation stone was laid by the Right Honourable Walter Long M.P.[11] on 27 July 1903, the then President of the Local Government Board in Balfour's Cabinet and who later became Chief Secretary for Ireland in March 1905. Although there were no houses around the Hammersmith Infirmary there had been a significant change in population between the census of 1871 and 1901. By 1901 the population of urban districts of England and Wales was over 77% of the whole, and that of rural districts a mere 23% (almost a reversal of the century before), yet the general population had increased by over 40%. The White City Stadium was erected in 1906[12] but the housing estate not until after the Great War.

THE PRISON

The Hospital was built next door to, but separated by a narrow road called Artillery Lane from, the walled prison of Wormwood Scrubs. When Millbank Prison, a national penitentiary in Pimlico, was condemned the Director of Convict Prisons bought 20 acres of land near the village of East Acton from the Ecclesiastical Commissioners: the deal was completed on 19 March 1874 for £10,019. On 14 December nine special-class prisoners moved into huts on the site to build accommodation for about 200 convict labourers. It was a severe winter and at times sledges were used across the snow to bring materials from the nearest railway station at Wood Lane and hence the first wing of the permanent prison was not even started until 8 August 1875. The man in charge was Major-General Edmund Du Cane, formerly of the Royal Engineers and a previous Inspector-General of Military Prisons. He later became Chairman of the Prison Commissioners to administer the Prison Act of 1877 (which nationalized the prisons and relieved boroughs of their costs) and was knighted the same year.

Du Cane was the chief architect of Wormwood Scrubs and, having been organizer of convict labour in Australia from 1851 to 1856, insisted that the Scrubs could be built more cheaply by convict labour: the cost per cell worked out at £70 compared with £130 to £198 at other prisons. He recognized in 1875 that the priority was 'to construct a good, hard track or roadway to Wood Lane. This took 1,863 cubic yards of brick ballast excavated and burnt for the purpose, and the track measured 920 yards.' The boundary wall was not completed until 1883 and all the original buildings, including a large and much admired Anglican chapel, by 1887. Sir Edmund Du Cane died in 1903, the year Walter Long laid the foundation stone of Hammersmith Hospital. His excellent water colours have been forgotten, but his suggestion of registration of criminals by composite portraits is still in use, and Du Cane Road, named after him, is a busy thoroughfare which also provides street parking for prison warders and hospital visitors.

Meanwhile golf had been introduced into the area by the formation of the Acton Golf Club in 1896 (part of the 'course' is now the A40 motorway). Indeed, in those days golf could be played from Shepherd's Bush to Harrow, without hindrance, on a series of five golf courses: the only one to remain today is at Sudbury. From the Hospital there was a clear view to Wood Lane until the White City Stadium was built. Originally the Olympic Games of 1908 were to be held in Rome, but in 1906 Mount Vesuvius erupted and this major catastrophe forced Italy to abandon the idea of acting as host nation to the games. Although this left very little time for any other country to build a stadium and living quarters for the competitors, and to organize transport and the events, Britain volunteered to do so. In less than 2 years the accommodation was completed and the Olympic Games opened at White City on 13 July 1908. In 1919 the 59 acres that formed the Acton Golf Club – the Hammersmith Infirmary was at its north-east border – were acquired by compulsory purchase order, and the land was developed that same year. Within a few years the three villages of Town Acton, Church Acton and East Acton, together with Ealing Village, Wembley and Harrow, were united by houses although all the land between them had originally been part of the green belt around London.

In 1928 a new St Clement Danes School was built on land alongside the Infirmary and to the east of it. Founded in 1862 as a church grammar school for boys in Holborn it had steadily grown in size and reputation. The site on which it stood in central London was valuable and the Church of England Commissioners decided to build a new and larger school on land owned by them at the corner of Du Cane Road and Scrubs Lane. The large sports field in the boys' school became a convenient landing ground for helicopters transporting patients from afar to the renal dialysis unit at Hammersmith. The patients used to be transferred to an ambulance and with police car escort, driven out of one entrance (the school) into the next (the hospital) even though there was a door in the wall separating the two establishments.

Hammersmith Hospital always had a close relationship with the prison: geographically, because they were next door to each other and at one time the only two buildings for miles around; socially, because the new nurses' home overlooked the prison and, particularly in summertime, the occupants of the former left their windows wide open and their radios full on for the benefit of the latter; professionally because many of the prisoners were attended by medical staff and occasionally used the Hospital premises as a route for escape. It was the flight of the spy Blake and his emigration to Russia in 1966 which put an end to fraternization and the introduction of special security by Lord Mountbatten. Hammersmith Hospital was sometimes referred to, in an affectionate sort of way, as 'St Wormwoods'. They have two features in common after 80 years of association; shortage of accommodation and shortage of car parking. Both appear insoluble.

THE HOSPITAL

The Board of Guardians new site was over 14 acres. The frontage was the Infirmary built along conventional lines: a long central corridor running parallel to the road with ward blocks across this at intervals. Behind the Infirmary, of similar design and parallel to it, but separated by an internal road, was the Workhouse. Both were built of the more expensive red brick, instead of the usual yellow, and pitched roofs of grey slate.

The completed building was formally opened by Her Royal Highness Princess Henry of Battenberg (the youngest of Queen Victoria's children) on 5 December 1905, and the new Hammersmith Infirmary attracted widespread interest, being regarded as too lavish and too costly. The buildings had cost £261,000, a very large sum, while the equipment was described as 'sumptuous'. The entrance hall was paved with mosaic (it still remains so) and surrounded by a dado of most expensive tiles (since painted over as a form of 'modernization'), while the dining hall was described as 'baronial splendour' and the Institution and Infirmary were often called the 'Pauper's Paradise' or the 'Palace on the Scrubs'. To the Victorian moralist the whole scheme must have appeared offensive, and a national newspaper editorial commented: 'Poverty is no longer a crime; 'tis not a fate to dread, but a circumstance to welcome. Spendthrift Guardians in contributing to pauperism, have robbed it of all its terrors – for Hammersmith, at least – and one may have no fear but that, when the time cometh, he may retire into quarters luxuriously finished and furnished, replete with every modern convenience as the auctioneer would say, and nearly as desirable, from the "Casuals" point of view, as that earlier institution which stands next door to Hammersmith's palace for the poor on Wormwood Scrubs.' The words of an outraged writer, but for the 'casual' it meant simply that he could do his work penance for a bed for the night under better conditions. As late as 1970 'the old labour yard' was a recognized geographical location between the two buildings. The North Block, which was the 'institution' was under a 'Master', Mr Andrews, and the South Block, the 'Infirmary' was under Dr John Jenkins, the Medical Superintendent.[13] Another writer had a more balanced view: 'These buildings combine the most recent improvements, and they are the latest advance in design, construction, and administrative detail. The Infirmary has been designed to provide accommodation for 330 sick persons, and the workhouse for 428 destitute poor. The Infirmary blocks are divided into wards, each of which will contain 34 beds, in addition to which there are the necessary administrative departments and a separate nurses' home, especially designed for the accommodation of an ample nursing staff. A completely equipped training school for nurses will be found in the Infirmary, in which the nursing staff will receive instruction in the theory and practice of their profession.'

Never before had Guardians spent so much on hospital and institutional provision, but undoubtedly Hammersmith was a great advance on the Poor Law hospitals of the time. Because it was better equipped and had better-trained nurses and doctors[14] it was able to treat the sick to standards comparable with those in the London voluntary hospitals. Nurse training started immediately: new nurses learnt from a senior nurse by an apprenticeship system. The nurse's day was from 7 a.m. to 8.30 p.m. with half-hourly breaks for meals thrice daily: there was 1 day off-duty each week, and later some off-duty time during the day. Most of the patients were long-stay, suffering from chronic or terminal diseases, and made heavy demands on nursing care. Indeed, most patients were admitted for nursing rather than medical care: there was no out-patient department and it was the medical superintendent who admitted all patients.

The usual salary of a Ward Sister was £36 a year plus board and lodging. The 10-bedded maternity unit had been approved for midwifery training by the new Central Midwives Board in 1906. In that year 30 probationers entered as nurse trainees. Indeed the total complement of 41 Hammersmith nurses[15] was made up of 10 trained nurses, 30 probationers, and one Receiving Ward nurse, yet the new Infirmary had 12 wards of 330 beds! All the nurses were accommodated in the nurses' home close to the main road, each nurse having a separate bedroom, a revolutionary step in those days. The Hammersmith soon became recognized as a first-rate training school: there was a carefully planned syllabus, similar to that of the General Nursing Council's of today, but more limited in scope. Lectures were given by the Medical Officers and by the Matron; practical instruction was provided by the Assistant Matron and Ward Sisters. On 9 November 1910 Miss Mary Northover, who had trained at the Middlesex Hospital, was appointed Matron and held that post until she retired in 1937 (she was succeeded by Miss Florence Campbell). In 1911 the total number of nurses was increased to 60 but conditions were still arduous: Day Sisters were required to relieve Night Sisters for 1 night each week and Night Nurses, who worked from 8 p.m. until 7 a.m., were allowed only 1 night off-duty each week.

By the outbreak of war in 1914, Hammersmith Infirmary was one of the most modern and best-equipped hospitals in the London area: wards had already been separated for medical, surgical, isolation, plaster, tuberculosis, children and maternity cases. Probably for these reasons the War Office took over the Hospital for the reception and treatment of wounded soldiers in 1915. In the Great War there were virtually no civilian casualties treated in hospitals in Britain, but many military were evacuated from the fighting in France (almost the complete reversal of what was to occur in the Second World War).

THE SHEPHERD'S BUSH

Early in 1916 Sir Robert Jones had been appointed by the War Office as Inspector of Military Orthopaedics. Now, Jones was the nephew of Hugh Owen Thomas, a famous orthopaedic surgeon of the last century, the inventor of the splint which bears his name and which today is still carried as standard equipment in ambulances and casualty units. In his memoirs he was later to write: 'The Great War afforded the most convincing proof of the mishandling of complicated, and even of simple, fractures. Fractures of the femur serve as a notable example. The splint with which we are all so familiar, invented by Thomas, was barely known, yet it was the type of splint which ultimately saved the situation. In 1916, the mortality from these fractures amounted to 80%, a large proportion of the deaths occurring on their way to or at the casualty clearning stations. Later when the Thomas splint was applied almost exclusively and as near to the firing line as possible, the mortality in 1918 was reduced to 20%.' (Thomas had previously offered his splint to the French during the war of 1870 and was rejected: he died in 1891.)

The army tradition was that in all military hospitals patients should be 'evacuated' to hospitals further from the acute zone as soon as they could be moved, so as to make room for more wounded. This continual transfer from one hospital to the next meant that with every move patients came under the care of a different surgeon. Moreover, a soldier had to be discharged from the Army as soon as it was clear that he would never be fit again for Army life. Jones held a meeting of orthopaedic surgeons to get agreement that there should be established a number of military orthopaedic hospitals – both in France and in England – where the wounded would stay until they were either fit to return to an Army unit or to be discharged from the Service: those returned to civilian life were to be taught a craft or trade before discharge, so that they could earn their living as civilians.

Jones then wrote to the Director General, Army Medical Services, Sir Alfred Keogh, pointing out that there was 'no systematic supervision of orthopaedic cases by men of special knowledge, that there was no cohesion between the various departments of treatment, such as massage, physical exercises, electricity, manipulative and operative groups of cases, all of which, properly controlled, make for success in orthopaedic surgery'. Finally Jones wrote: 'It appears to me that we want one large orthopaedic hospital combining all these departments and staffed by men under a director, who should be the final arbiter of treatment. This hospital should contain at least 800 beds and should be a military hospital.'

Keogh agreed to these revolutionary but logical ideas and the War Office asked the Board of Guardians for the use of Hammersmith Infirmary and Institution for this purpose. The Guardians agreed, the patients and inmates were transferred elsewhere, and in February 1916 the buildings became the 'Military Orthopaedic Hospital, Shepherd's Bush'. Although Hammersmith contained the 800 beds required, these were not enough: as many as 200 patients were billeted locally in requisitioned houses, attending the Hospital daily. Jones' ideas were approved by such surgeons as Moynihan (20 years later to become a Governor of the British Postgraduate Medical School) and Stiles. The Red Cross Society supported the Hospital and Queen Alexandra visited it in 1917.

Jones soon collected a brilliant group of surgeons to work there: Aitken, Dunn, Emslie, Bristow, Evans, Barkart, Wood Jones, Trethowan, Verrall, and Sir Thomas Dunhill. Practically every eminent orthopaedic surgeon of the interwar years had worked at 'Shepherd's Bush', and many of the names are familiar in that specialty today. The Commanding Officers were John Jenkins (the former Medical Superintendent, who therefore knew the Hospital intimately), Walter Hill and later Picton Phillips. Curative workshops were built and about half of the 800 patients were being trained or employed in them. The effect on the morale of the patients was enormous and 'Shepherd's Bush' became the prototype of many other military hospitals in the provinces. Watson,[16] said that 'The historical importance of "Shepherd's Bush" is that it became the first experimental hospital in training the disabled.'

Jones' philosophy was simple: he understood the motivation and drive necessary for successful rehabilitation. In the preface to his book, *Notes on Military Orthopaedics* (1916), he wrote: 'Men with stiff ankles are set to drive a treadle, lathe or fretsaw. If put on a treadle-exercising machine the monotony soon wearies the mind, but if the mind is engaged not on the monotony of the footwork, but on the interest of the work turned out, neither mind nor body becomes tired.' And again about rehabilitation after discharge from the Army: 'If I were wounded and received a full pension of 25/– a week, and was asked to learn a trade by which I could make 15/– and be paid 10/– pension I should probably prefer to remain idle. [A sentiment currently still used about unemployment benefit.] The discharged soldier should have every incentive to work, so that his industry should add to his wealth. The productivity of his labour becomes the important asset to the Nation, not the number of shillings paid out to him.'

The first experimental rehabilitation workshop was opened at 'Shepherd's Bush' on 1 March 1916, and in the same month Robert Jones was appointed Inspector of Military Orthopaedics. He was now authorized to establish orthopaedic hospitals upon the same principles as 'Shepherd's Bush' in other parts of Great Britain: he did so at Manchester, Leeds, Newcastle, Oxford, Reading, Cardiff, Birmingham, Bristol, Bath, Edinburgh, Glasgow, Aberdeen, Dublin and Belfast. Jones hoped that as 'Shepherd's Bush' gathered about it a tradition, it might with a little imagination have become a permanent national institution: 'instead of which it was ordained by some inscrutable fate that it should arise from the mediocrity of a Poor House, and to that forlorn destiny return'. For several years the exiled King Manoel of Portugal worked at 'Shepherd's Bush', from early morning till late evening. simply and solely for the cause of the disabled. He raised large sums of money by public appeal and was the representative of the Red Cross there. 'Shepherd's Bush' created more interest and aroused more enthusiasm than any other hospital during the war. Many American surgeons came to work there in 1917: indeed during the Great War both Plastic Surgery and Orthopaedic Surgery had a high proportion of U.S.A. surgeons in U.K. hospitals.

Watson wrote that 'Shepherd's Bush' was not only a great military hospital for the wounded soldier during the war, but for the pensioner after the armistice. It lay at the heart of two signal contributions to war and peace. It demonstrated the possibilities of orthopaedic surgery in the greatest city in the world and it preached the gospel of rehabilitation. As Jones himself said in 1917 – he was knighted that year – 'I have lived and worked long enough to realise that the aim and not the end is the main thing.'

In March 1919, 'Shepherd's Bush' was still under the War Office, but during the summer it was taken over by the Ministry of Pensions who rented it for £8000 a year. The Red Cross bequeathed their equipment to the Ministry, and King Manuel resigned with some bitterness, although he did receive a letter of appreciation from General Sir John Goodwin for his 'services for the wounded soldier'. The final struggle to preserve 'Shepherd's Bush' for the nation came in February 1922. Jones wrote a letter to *The Times* newspaper: 'For its unique equipment and admirable staff work, "Shepherd's Bush", as a pioneer of recent orthopaedic surgery and for its continued post-war activity, has been recognised not only by the medical world as a distinguished centre, but to the men themselves, wherever they may be, as a city of refuge when hope of recovery grows faint.' But it was no use. This model hospital 'was fated to be handed back to a body of Guardians for a purpose as dreary as it was insignificant'. To him this action was preposterous. The hospital was released by the Pensions Ministry on 11 April 1925, and 9 years' history in military orthopaedics was terminated. Sir Robert Jones died on 14 January 1933, a recognized leader in his specialty and the first President of the International Society of Orthopaedics.

With the return of their hospital the Guardians continued to provide first-class medical treatment. Jenkins returned as Medical Superintendent and Miss Northover as Matron. A new consultant staff was appointed, including Fedden, Rocyn Jones, Torrens, Slot, Loughnane, Cecil Wakeley, Williamson-Noble and Winsbury-White – the last three to become very well known and to write textbooks. When the hospital was transferred to the London County Council on 1 April 1930, more staff were appointed: Ivor Griffiths (E.N.T.), Sir Harold Gillies and Pomfret Kilner (Plastic Surgery), G. W. Theobald (Gynaecology) and Francis Walshe (Neurology). The Infirmary and Institution were merged, the nursing staff was increased to 200 and a qualified Sister Tutor appointed. By 1931 the Chamberlain–Greenwood Committee had decided that Hammersmith should become the University Postgraduate Hospital and have attached to it the British Postgraduate Medical School, and thus implement the recommendations of the Athlone Committee.

The First World War produced two important and practical medical advances: organized orthopaedics (at the 'Shepherd's Bush') and the specialty of Plastic Surgery (originally at Sidcup, later moved to the 'Shepherd's Bush' at the end of the war before transferring to Roehampton). Interestingly the provisional organization of the Postgraduate Medical Education Committee of 1930 (Appendix A) showed a scheme for the future Hospital Service: the Surgical Division included Orthopaedics and Plastic Surgery, yet within that decade Orthopaedics was to expand and Plastic Surgery to become almost extinct. In the past 50 years the Hammersmith has never had a Professor of Orthopaedics, but did appoint a Professor of Plastic and Reconstructive Surgery in 1970. By 1980 there were 20 Professors of Orthopaedics in Britain, but only one Professor of Plastic Surgery.

4

The Birth of the Postgraduate Medical School

The first meeting of the 'Governors-Designate of the School and others interested in the work of the School' was held on 3 June 1931 with Lord Chelmsford in the chair: a Planning and Building Sub-committee was also set up, and met 2 weeks later on 17 June 1931. On 10 July 1931 a Royal Charter was granted, confirming those already in office and allowing co-option. The first meeting of the Governing Body proper took place on 15 July 1931 and co-opted Webb-Johnson (later to become President of the Royal College of Surgeons), Menzies (Medical Officer of Health for the County Council of London), and Dr Louisa Martindale.

The Treasury and the London County Council (L.C.C.) had each agreed to provide £250,000 for the new buildings and their equipment: plans had been prepared to spend this sum on new laboratories, school buildings, an operating theatre, out-patient department, and improvement to the wards. In September 1931 a national financial crisis occurred which nearly caused the whole scheme to be abandoned: the first reaction of the Treasury and the L.C.C. was exactly that. However, Lord Chelmsford and Sir Allen Daley[17] saw Sir Arthur Robinson (Secretary to the Treasury) to ask for further consideration, but it was really Sir Frederick Menzies, Medical Officer of the L.C.C., whose persuasion enabled a start to be made on the proposed school. He first saw Sir Angus Scott, Chairman of the L.C.C. Finance Committee, and persuaded him to put up £100,000 for the scheme if the Treasury would match it: Scott agreed.

Menzies then saw Neville Chamberlain, now back as Minister of Health, to ask him to persuade the Chancellor of the Exchequer, Philip Snowden, to put up £100,000 if the L.C.C. would match it! Snowden, convinced that the other side would never accept, agreed to find that sum. When Menzies put the two notes that he had got them to write in front of Sir Angus Scott, he was called rude names but told: 'Go ahead. You shall have your money and you deserve it.' Both sides kept their promises and a joint expenditure of £200,000 was authorized. Naturally, the original building plans had to be drastically cut, but a start could be made. Indeed, the building trade was short of work and such favourable tenders were received that more could be spent on equipment than expected.

The government crisis was not purely financial but political too. The great economic Depression broke world-wide on 29 October 1929 when the speculative Bubble burst in the U.S.A. and American money ceased to flow, particularly to Great Britain. Primary producers no longer wanted to buy British ships and declined British money. As a result the exporters, already in difficulties, saw their remaining markets disappear and unemployment rose rapidly. By July 1930 there were over 2 million unemployed, and 2½ million in December: 3 million were expected, incorrectly, for 1931. In the event the figure fell, the volume of imports remained stable, and with the fall in prices the value of wages rose.

Snowden's budget for 1930 increased income tax to four shillings and sixpence in the pound, but by 1931 the yield from taxes had gone down, so a cut in unemployment benefits was planned and opposition to MacDonald's Government became manifest. As a result, MacDonald's First National Government was formed in August.

The second meeting of the Governing Body was held on 15 October 1931, when members learnt of the compromise (they would have £200,000 and not the ½ million pounds expected) and the third on 4 December 1931. The post of Dean was to be advertised, with the following requirements.

The Dean will[18]:

1. be principal executive officer of the Governing Body,
2. arrange students courses,
3. be responsible for the administrative and financial management of the school,
4. be required to undergo a medical examination before appointment and will normally retire at the age of 60,
5. attend every subcommittee,
6. report the names of officers absent from duty,
7. prepare the annual estimates, and
8. interview students, but 'this memorandum does not purport to be exhaustive'.

He was to be paid £2000 annually and debarred from private practice in this full-time post. The salary was a large sum in those days and drew a smart response from the Treasury official, Mr Stocks, who wrote: 'the advertisement suggests that you are looking for a man who is going to take on himself the function of advertising agent, principal executive officer, director of studies and chief accountant as well as give lectures of a high standard. How far do the Committee really expect the Dean to perform all these duties himself? Do they contemplate as a definite administrative establishment only the Dean with a clerk and shorthand typist. . . . other schools have generally found it necessary to have a responsible officer besides the Dean . . . are you clear that such an appointment is not likely to be required here? We only raise this point now because in similar cases we have been landed with an expensive Dean at the start, only to find later that a humbler man is wanted to do most of his work and that the Dean himself can be a part-time officer with a nominal salary, and is more efficient.' The letter ends: 'The Committee will, of course, already have thought all this out, and we should like to know at this stage what is their idea of the organism to be and how far its life will depend on the Dean's personal labours.'

This was a fairly sarcastic letter and the Governing Body took no notice of the advice, although the advertisement was held up. The Treasury took strong exception to a salary of £2000 being offered. Lord Chelmsford personally went to the Treasury and was able to compromise on a figure of £1800 inclusive.

A PERIOD OF UNCERTAINTY

The Committee met only once in 1932, on 29 January, at which detailed architects' plans were considered. It was already clear that Sir Frederick Menzies and Lord Dawson of Penn were the two most determined members to get the building under way. In that year there was still high unemployment, political instability (MacDonald's National Government), continuing financial crises, a drift away from the conventional heavy industries into newer lines, buses carried more passengers than trams, and despite a Royal Charter there seemed good reason to believe that the British Postgraduate Medical School would never materialize. The budget of April 1932 heralded lean times but recovery from the great Depression began the following year, so that by 1937 production and employment were at peak levels. According to Professor Harrison,[19] the architects were given three pieces of information – all three incorrect – and probably by Professor Dean, a co-opted member who was Professor of Pathology at Cambridge. First, all laboratories need a north light – based on the assumption that microscopes used daylight for illumination, although by that time most were in fact using artificial light – so that all windows were to face north where possible. Second, all benches were standing benches, 36 inches high. Third, all clinicians work at the bedside (the word clinic being derived from the Greek word for a bed) and so do not need labs or offices. Harrison wrote that the first did not matter, the second was a nuisance and some benches were lowered but most adopted the high stool to sit, but the third was a major catastrophe: 'when the clinical professors arrived they had no rooms to sit in'. As a result, a hut was hastily erected between L block and B block (the wooden building is still in use, named 'Lower Medical Corridor' to distinguish it from the laboratories on the top of L block) and accommodated all clinical staff until the end of the war. But in effect the appointment of a Dean and the start of building were both deferred. Interestingly there were 70 enquiries for the post of Dean, and 15 applications, of which two were estimated to be of outstanding merit.

The meeting on 7 February 1933 was chaired by Sir Austen Chamberlain, Lord Chelmsford having resigned and become Warden of All Souls, Oxford (he died on 1 April 1933). At this meeting a draft agreement was drawn up, of 29 pages, prepared by the L.C.C. solicitors, which defined what hospital alterations would be carried out, who would pay and how, maintenance of equipment, nominations of resident practitioners, nursing staff, and a great deal more. In effect, this 1933 Agreement meant that the School was required to pay the L.C.C. for any extra expenditure on medical services resulting from the affiliation of the Hospital with the School. It was inevitable, expected, and no doubt predicted, that standards were going to be raised and the School would have to pay the difference. Later, Sir John McMichael[20] was to refer to the 'iniquity' of such an agreement, and that the bill was never paid – nor could it have been – because the sum was about £50,000 in 1939 when war started: in his own words, the bill was 'quietly forgotten' (but in fact it was paid, as the audited accounts show, and a sum of £5000 annually until the advent of the N.H.S. in 1948). On 19 May 1933 Sir Frederick Menzies was able to report that the L.C.C. had accepted the lowest tender for building and that the Medical School might be finished before the academic year, beginning October 1934. The foundation stone was laid by Mr Neville Chamberlain, by then Chancellor of the Exchequer, on 7 July 1933. Six hundred and forty distinguished guests were invited: prayers were said before the speeches, a band and three trumpeters sounded a fanfare after the stone was laid (the stone can be seen to the left of the entrance to the Shah Lecture theatre at about eye level). An editorial in *The Times* of 14 July 1933 said: 'The Chancellor of the Exchequer and the Chairman of the Governors of the School are, not improbably, helping to forward today a development no less momentous for the health and happiness of peoples remote as well as near than the organisation for the study and treatment of tropical diseases created by the vision and force of their father at the Colonial Office nearly 40 years ago' (a reference to the School of Hygiene and Tropical Medicine, founded 1929). Sir Austen Chamberlain was the Chairman of the Board of Governors: the Earl of Athlone, whose committee had recommended the founding of the School of Tropical Medicine and the Postgraduate Medical School, was present with the Minister of Health, Sir Hilton Young. The building planned for the School was to be of 'three stories arranged round a square courtyard, thus providing abundant light and ventilation'. The 'clinical theatre' was large enough to accommodate 'close on 100 students': above this there was a larger lecture theatre and over the School Offices 'a well lit library and two rooms for the teaching staff'.

The building had cost £46,000 and left a balance of £35,000 for equipment, well within the allowed budget: the hospital building costs were similarly arranged.

RECRUITMENT OF STAFF

At the next meeting of Governors on 16 October 1934, Sir Edwin Deller (Principal of the University of London) was present by invitation. He gave advice on the appointment of a Dean and offered three alternatives: a layman, a doctor who could if necessary be one of the four foundation professors already agreed on, or a doctor who was primarily an administrator but who also held a part-time non-professorial post on the teaching staff of the School (the last was favoured by the Committee, and this had also been the view at the meeting in December 1931). At the interview 2 weeks after, Dr Malcolm Henry MacKeith[21] was appointed Dean to take office on 1 January 1934; he was 38, had trained at Guy's and was a Demonstrator in Pharmacology and Dean of the Medical School at the University of Oxford. Automatically he became a Governor and attended the next meeting, to select the Professors.

Lord Dawson put the case for allowing professors to have limited private practice, arguing that a professor would not be a good teacher if his clinical experience was limited to hospital patients. Dr Barrie Lambert countered this argument: 'Was not the real object of the proposed innovation to increase the income of the professor?' In the end, 'it was agreed that the salary of the three clinical professors should be £2500 per annum,[22] and the salary of the Professor of Pathology £2000'. Moreover, 'the number of beds under the direct control of the professor will never be less than fifty'. Each professor and all members of his staff would be 'approved and individually appointed as members of the L.C.C. hospital staff' and paid by means of a bock grant annually by the L.C.C. But the University of London had yet to aprove the whole venture. The Finance and General Purposes Committee prepared an estimate of the maintenance costs to submit to the University Grants Committee, and the Governors set up a Board of Advisers to appoint the professors. They were Sir Austen Chamberlain (Chairman), Sir Frederick Menzies (L.C.C.), Lord Dawson of Penn (Medicine), Professor Gask (Surgery), Dr Watts Eden (Obstetrics and Gynaecology) and Professor Dean (Pathology).

The Dean, Dr MacKeith, as Secretary to the Governors and replacing Mr North, an officer of the Ministry of Health (who had acted as secretary to the Committee until then), made two serious mistakes. The first was in his estimates submitted on 9 January 1934 to the University Grants Committee: the estimated expenditure, because the School was unlikely to open before October 1934, was £20,330 for the salaries for the four Professors and their four Readers so that posts could be advertised immediately, but a special committee of the Governors now decided that the Department of Pathology should include three main subjects – morbid anatomy, pathological chemistry and bacteriology – all under the direction of one Professor, each requiring a person of the standing of a Reader to be in charge. Nine days later, Dr MacKeith had to send a second letter to the University Grants Committee with a revised estimate but only for two Readers in Pathology and not the three required. The parent body, the Treasury, did not reply in time for the professorships to be advertised by the end of January, as had been hoped, although by then it was obvious that the building work would not be completed before December.

The Lords Commissioners of His Majesty's Treasury wrote on 27 February that they were not pleased that each of the clinical professors was to be paid a salary of £2500 – 'the standard of remuneration would appear to be considerably more expensive than that in force in other medical and scientific schools in this country' – but, after considerable hesitation, felt able to accept the conclusion that the 'exceptional importance of these posts in the medical teaching world must be marked by a financial standing superior to that of comparable posts in other schools', etc. and so they approved the salaries. The Reader's salary was to be £1000. They also wished to know what contribution the London County Council was going to make towards the consultants' salaries.

The second mistake was also to do with the Readers. The Dean was not familiar with the machinery of the university and discovered by chance that the university had to establish the post of Readership before a Reader could be appointed. This matter was resolved in September 1934. The University of London announced in February 1934 its 'recognition' of the new institution as a school of that university, and also approved certain proposals regarding the conditions of tenure of the Professors. At the meeting of 8 June 1934, the Governing Body approved the appointments of:

Professor F. R. Fraser to the Chair of Medicine.[23]
Professor James Young to the Chair of Midwifery.[24]
Professor E. H. Kettle to the Chair of Pathology.[25]

At the same meeting Paymaster Captain W. R. Scotland R.N. was appointed personal assistant to the Dean (a post later to be known as School Secretary). Professor Wilkie had evidently declined the Chair of Surgery (he was after all comfortably ensconced in Edinburgh as Professor and Senior Surgeon), and it was proposed to invite Professor Grey Turner[26] of Newcastle on Tyne to accept the post: he accepted but could not take up his duties until 1935.

However, he was present with the other Professors at the first meeting of the School Council (later to be called the Academic Board) on 24 July 1934.

Under the School Charter the Council could have contained at least 18 members. The Governing Body decided to keep it small – wisely, because there was a lot of business to get through and in the event it had to meet fortnightly, sometimes weekly, and appointed the following: Lord Dawson of Penn, Mr Eason and Professor Gask (these three to represent the Governing Body), the Dean, the four professors, and Sir Frederick Menzies (Chief Medical Officer of the London County Council). Captain Scotland and Sir Thomas Carey Evans (an ex-Indian Medical Service doctor who had been appointed Medical Superintendent to the hospital) attended by invitation. Professor Gask was to act as Chairman until October 1935 and there were no formal standing orders. The organization and staffing of the four departments were agreed. The Board of Advisers recommended the following appointments:

Reader in Obstetrics and Gynaecology, Dr J. C. Moir,[27] as from 1 December 1934.
Reader in Medicine, Dr R. S. Aitkin,[28] as from 1 January 1935.
Reader in Surgery, Mr L. C. Rogers,[29] as from 1 January 1935.
Reader in Pathological Chemistry, Dr E. J. King,[30] as from 1 January 1935.
Reader in Bacteriology, Dr A. A. Miles,[31] as from 1 January 1935.

Within 10 years all had become professors themselves: only Professor Earl King remained with the school. At the meeting of the Governing Body on 19 October 1934 the above appointments were ratified and the university informed. Dr MacKeith, the Dean, tendered his resignation on the grounds of ill-health to take effect from 31 December 1934. Colonel A. H. Proctor D.S.O., M.D., F.R.C.S., who had been in the Indian Medical Service all his life and who at 55 did not measure up to the original specifications detailed in 1931, was appointed Dean on 18 January 1935 and took up his appointment on 1 February. Presumably, the other 'outstanding candidate' on the short list in 1934, Dr A. E. Clark-Kennedy, did not apply: he was by then in line to be Dean of the London Hospital Medical School, a post he held with distinction for 17 years and retired in 1953. Colonel Proctor never really fitted in with the life of a University School and Hospital although he worked in complete harmony with the Medical Superintendent of the Hospital (they were both I.M.S.): in 1939 he became Commandant of a wartime military hospital (where he was immensely popular), never to return.

The School was fortunate to have a man of the eminence of Sir Austen Chamberlain as Chairman of the Governing Body: he was already 71 and was still Chairman when he died in 1937. Sir Austen, half-brother of the younger Mr Neville Chamberlain, had twice been Chancellor of the Exchequer, Foreign Secretary, and twice declined the post of Prime Minister. For the School estimates of 1935/1936 he corresponded personally with Mr J. A.

Barlow at the Treasury. As a result a grant-in-aid of £36,000 was awarded, and the Governing Body congratulated Sir Austen on the 'bargain he had concluded' and that the Treasury had recognized the 'importance of the School'. The new buildings were completed just after Christmas 1934, and were occupied piecemeal in January and February 1935, a procedure of occupation by osmosis that was to be repeated 20 years later in the new medical school known as the Commonwealth Building. Mr G. A. Lloyd, aged 23, was appointed Librarian at a salary of £250 per annum, just one-tenth of that of a clinical professor, but £1000 was included in the estimates for books and journals. The library was housed on the first floor of L block on the west side, later to become the main teaching laboratory for the Diploma in Clinical Pathology Course.

THE FORMAL OPENING

The School was formally declared open by His Majesty King George V on 13 May 1935. For the King it may have been a tiring day (he died in January the following year) but for everyone else it was the practical realization of a dream going back two decades. In his address at the opening of the British Postgraduate Medical School, King George V said: 'It is my earnest hope that this School, with its happy union of ward and laboratory, University and Local Authority, drawing students from all parts of our Empire, and, I trust, from regions even more widely spread, may prosper under God's blessing. May it play an imperial role in the relief of suffering among my peoples in this country and overseas, and in enabling the doctors of all lands to come together in a task where all must be allies and helpers.' At last, after 10 years of dreaming and planning, the School was a reality. It now had to demonstrate its worth, and that its impeccable pedigree meant great things ahead.

5

Infancy and War

The first student was enrolled on 13 May 1935. Between then and 31 July 1936 there were 525 students of whom 310 came from various parts of Britain and the remaining 40% from different countries, including India 74, South Africa 33, Canada 25 and Australia 21. The Annual Report for 1936 set out the objectives of the School in these words: 'the School has been established to provide instruction for qualified medical practitioners only. No undergraduates are admitted, and with a few exceptions no courses are organised with a view to preparing candidates for higher degrees or diplomas. Excellent courses for these degrees and diplomas are already available at the undergraduate schools. The work of the School is arranged to provide for –

(a) Medical practitioners who are prepared to spend any period from one month to a year in improving their knowledge.
(b) Officers of the medical services of the Crown specialising in any branch of Medicine.
(c) Intensive Refresher Courses for general practitioners designed to bring before them recent advances in subjects of special interest to them.
(d) Similar courses spread over a longer period for general practitioners with a small amount of spare time available.
(e) Lectures and demonstrations by recognized authorities on the subjects they will deal with.
(f) Research work by the Staff and facilities for research by students under proper supervision.'

The same report mentioned the Association with Hammersmith Hospital (L.C.C.): 'The number and variety of cases admitted to the Hospital has been adequate for the purpose of the School, and the general conditions well suited to teaching. The London County Council have provided new wards, operation theatres, and a well-equipped radiological and out-patient department to meet the special requirements. Further extensions are in progress.'

The 1936 Report was too optimistic. Although the School had been a success from the start, it was never founded or funded in the way that was originally intended. Both School and Hospital have suffered from chronic shortage of funds ever since that cut in allocation in 1931; by 1938 the School was in serious need of additional buildings, but preparations for war put a stop to any further expansion. The 1933 Agreement had set out the respective responsibilities of School and Hospital: in essence the London County Council was responsible for the care of patients and administration of the hospital, the School for teaching and research although the staff of the School was given charge of the beds.

SOME DEFICIENCIES

The British Postgraduate Medical School had only 4 years in which to develop some sort of strategy, before war came and the whole enterprise was in jeopardy. Having survived the war, the urgency then was to remedy two glaring defects of academic recognition, radiology and anaesthetics – neither of which had been debated by the Athlone nor the Chamberlain Committees, an extraordinary omission – both of which were necessary in a university hospital.

When the Würzburg Physical Medical Society on New Year's Day 1896 published Roentgen's paper 'On a new kind of rays: a preliminary communication', it not only broke with tradition that all papers had to be presented to the Society orally before publication (the *Proceedings of the Royal Society of Medicine of London* were so treated until recently) but also acknowledged the outstanding importance of Roentgen's discovery. The rest of the world agreed and by 1935 an X-ray machine had been installed in every hospital. At Hammersmith Hospital the radiologist was Dr E. J. E. Topham, the X-ray machine was next to the operating theatre on the ground floor between C and D blocks, but when the School was founded the London County Council built a new department in L block, decided that a more senior and experienced man was needed as Director and appointed Dr Duncan White who was in charge of diagnostic and therapeutic X-rays. He was appointed to teach and to develop the discipline. During the war he was a specialist in the army at Milbank with the rank of major until invalided out with clear evidence that he was suffering from the effects of radiation: this was to be the fate of many of the early pioneers, and White like them died of radiation-induced cancer.

In 1942 the Medical Research Council Radium Unit moved from Lambeth Hospital to Hammersmith when it was bombed during the 'blitz': the risk of keeping such valuable and dangerous material in central London was also appreciated. White accepted that radiotherapy would develop as a separate discipline under Dr Constance Wood who was housed on the second floor of L block above his own unit which was above the Out-patient Department, a building erected beside and at the same time as the School.

The four Foundation Professors used diagnostic radiology extensively and White was part of the new School in all but name. In 1946 Topham left and Steiner was appointed in his place but not until 1950. By 1953 White was seriously ill and resigned. Steiner alone had to manage the Department which had grown in size: in 1936 referrals for examination totalled 5386: in 1951 there were 26,000 and by 1980 over 50,000. The ancient equipment was replaced, new techniques were developed and others in the School (Aird, Goodwin, Harrison, Bewley, Fraser, Milne) began to appreciate what was on offer; joint publications appeared and an academic atmosphere enveloped this service department. John Laws[32] joined in 1955, Frank Doyle[33] later – both full-time N.H.S. appointments – and Steiner was made Professor of Diagnostic Radiology in 1961, a personal Chair later to be recognized as an established post. The Department had become part of the University Hospital and Medical School, but it had taken the best part of 20 years to accomplish. As it grew in importance, staff, and equipment there was nowhere to expand: in 1966 the angiographic unit slid into the old Lecture Theatre on the same floor, but space was a major problem for a discipline that clearly was developing rapidly. When the M.R.C. built a new unit for the cyclotron in the north-east corner of the site – to be a showpiece at the Queen's visit for the Hospital's Golden Jubilee in 1955 – the second floor of L block was retained for hospital radiotherapy. Hence it was not until 1983, after scanners had come into their own more than a decade before, that a grossly overcrowded Radiology Department could occupy the floor above and expand laterally over the area of an extended Out-patient Department. When Allison took over from Steiner he had acquired space, equipment, active collaborative research with almost every other academic department and the discipline of Radiology had changed out of all recognition: for clinicians it was as important as biochemistry in managing patients.

When the School was founded, most anaesthetics were given by general practitioners in cottage hospitals and by recently qualified doctors in teaching hospitals. Some London hospitals had appointed a consultant to the staff: at Hammersmith, Woodfield-Davies[36] and Rait-Smith[37] were the consultants to four surgeons in 1936 at a time when anaesthesia was mainly 'rag and bottle'. In 1950 a Department of Anaesthesia was created with two Lecturers (Smith and Hilda Roberts) and four part-time N.H.S. consultants (Dorothy Spence-Sales, Woodfield-Davies, Beard, and Wood-Smith): two more joined in 1959 (Lloyd-Jones and Nunn). It was not until 1964 that a Chair was created and a Professor appointed (J. G. Robson)[38] but by 1984 the Department had two Professors, three Senior Lecturers, four Honorary Senior Lecturers, and one sessional Senior Lecturer, a total of ten senior staff. By then too, anaesthetics had become the largest single specialty in Britain, and Hammersmith had provided seven of the twenty current Professors of Anaesthesia. Already there had begun to appear three distinct sub-specialties within the main discipline: intensive care, pharmacology, and pain relief, all with a spirit of scientific experiment and Ph.D. was becoming a necessary qualification for entry to the academic ranks, a situation that could not have been forecast half a century earlier.

THE DEVELOPMENT OF AN ETHOS

Sir John McMichael[39] has stated that the basic pattern for the School was set by Francis Fraser, the foundation Professor of Medicine: 'It was to be a university centre with whole-time academic staffing and with research opportunities for the staff.' There was agreement that only by pursuing research in his particular field of study could 'a specialist build an academic reputation, become expert in his subject, develop enthusiasm about his subject and transmit this enthusiasm to his juniors'. The qualified doctors, wishing to learn more, had to be taught by experts, never amateurs, and have readily available collateral experts: other institutes could, and did, concentrate on specialization based on diseases of a single system (they were united as the British Postgraduate Medical Federation in 1947), but not Hammersmith, which intended to remain as a general hospital.

Professor Kettle died on 1 December 1936, a heavy loss to the School: he was only 54 and had had little time to make his mark at the Hammersmith. He had been the Professor of Pathology at the Welsh National School of Medicine, then at Bart's before coming to Hammersmith:[40] he was succeeded by Professor Henry Dible who was 47 at the time, and the youngest of the four professors. All in all, 1936 was not a good year for Hammersmith or for the country. In March Hitler had reoccupied the demilitarized zone of the Rhineland, in May the Italians captured Addis Ababa, and King Victor Emmanual III of Italy was proclaimed Emperor of Abyssinia, the Spanish Civil War started – many Britons were to join the International Brigade, and to join Communism too, against Germany and Italy who supported Franco (whose final victory did not come until April 1939) – and Edward VIII abdicated, having been King for less than a year. By 1937 the pace of rearmament had become fast enough to affect the finances of the country, which was now committed to a £1500 million programme. Chamberlain imposed a tax on profits to pay for this, and when he formed his National Government in May 1937 Sir Kingsley Wood became Minister of Health, only to move to be Secretary for Air a year later (and he was to be replaced by Walter Elliott, the Secretary for Scotland). On 30 September 1938 Neville Chamberlain returned from his appeasement talks with Hitler at Munich ('Peace with honour') but rearmament continued. On 31 March 1939 Polish sovereignty was guaranteed and on 26 April conscription of 6 months duration was introduced for all men aged 20 and 21.

PREPARATION FOR WAR

In 1938 the whole of Europe was on the brink of war. When the subject was being debated in the House of Commons and Neville Chamberlain announced that he was to meet Mr Hitler at Munich next day, members from both sides of the House cheered with relief. The possibility of the Hospital being required to take air-raid casualties was considered at Hammersmith, and a scheme was prepared in which every member of staff was allotted specific duties, divided into night and day duties. This insured that the Hospital could be 'worked at its maximum capacity as regards operating theatres, reception rooms, resuscitation wards etc.'. The organization was not put to the test of actual casualties, although one suspects that some were keen to find out how good it really was, but a blood transfusion service was started. Special apparatus was designed by Dr Janet Vaughan (Senior Assistant in Clinical Pathology) to simplify the collection and administration of blood: in the event, Janet Vaughan organized the Blood Transfusion Service for north London and ran it effectively until 1944 when she became Principal of Somerville College, Oxford. She was also an ardent Socialist – interviewed on T.V. on 5 August 1984 – have seen and treated anaemia in the poverty around the London Hospital when all that was needed was good food.

The new Nurses' Home was opened in 1938 and the London County Council was asked to allow the old Nurses' Home to be used as a hostel for students, particularly obstetric students: in 1940 after war had started and many hospitals were evacuated from central London, undergraduates from St Mary's and the London Hospital[41] did their midwifery there. Later, in 1942, it was used for Canadian and U.S.A. doctors attending 'War Courses': again in 1945 it was used to accommodate Service doctors from Canada and the U.S.A. attending 6-week courses in midwifery before they went home and back to civilian life. Being together on site helped to provide some communal life for men who were strangers to London, and the L.C.C. was thanked for the generous action. As the Dean wrote in his Report: 'It was a temporary return to a sort of collegiate life which all doctors have experienced during their training, and which was all the more welcome after a period of life under Service conditions. The Canadians (and later the Americans) acquired a new opinion of the British as a result of this hospitality on the part of the London County Council'. The old Nurses' Home remains today as the resident doctors' quarters: from without, it appears unchanged from the day it was built 80 years ago: from within, modernization has brought the accommodation to the level of the average hostel for itinerants.

As Britain drifted to the war of 1939 the machinery and prestige of the

League of Nations was shattered, and the rulers of Italy, Germany and Japan proceeded with preparations for fresh conquests. At the Hammersmith there was little opportunity to move forward: in 1938 Europe was on the brink of war and spent that year expecting it. Hammersmith had the best of today's men who brought their wide experience, recognized authority and international reputation of their respective subjects, from publications and world-wide travel, to the School and Hospital to give both the status that was needed. But they could not bring youth. They were men wise in their ways and at the top of their profession, but they were old men: Fraser was 54, Turner 61, Young 56 and Dible 50. What Hammersmith needed was the best of tomorrow's men: they were waiting in the wings ready to come on stage when the chance arose.

When Churchill became leader of Britain and her Allies in May 1940 the spirit of the thirties died. Within weeks the evacuation of the British Forces from Dunkirk (26 May to 4 June 1940) made everyone aware of change. 'The essence of the spirit of the thirties was not apathy but inertia: a structural resistance to change and especially to any radical improvement . . . consciences were deeply stirred, but could find no outlet in constructive action. The sense of helplessness and drift that resulted may explain the escapist flavour of the most fashionable cults.'[42]

Until the outbreak of war the Hospital and School had developed together rapidly, increasing in fame and prestige. The war was a shattering blow. The postgraduates departed for sterner duties, the number of Hammersmith Hospital beds in active commission was reduced drastically – all top floor wards were evacuated – and the main operating theatres closed and transferred to the ground floor (there was no basement: several of London's hospitals transferred theatres to basements so that work could continue throughout air raids). Many of the medical staff and nurses were transferred to hospitals on the outskirts of London, and the future of the Hammersmith seemed uncertain: if it had been severely bombed it was unlikely to rise again, like a Phoenix from the ashes, and postgraduate medicine would have taken a different turning. Indeed the Dean at the time, Colonel Proctor, told the staff quite bluntly that the whole scheme should be dropped (he then departed to command a military hospital) which must have depressed everyone. Originally the School was responsible only for the 458 beds in the South Hospital: the more chronic cases in the North Hospital were under the sole care of the London County Council Staff. In 1939 it was agreed that the School should manage all 680 beds.

The Government experts had expected the Germans to drop 100,000 tons of bombs on London in 14 days – the total on London throughout the war never reached that figure – and they used a multiplier of 50 (that is, each one ton of bombs would cause 50 casualties). Each bomb was predicted to fall on a densely populated area and no 'misses' were allowed for. The actual multiplier in London turned out to be 15–20.[43] The experts, and the government for that matter, expected an air attack to last 60 days, leaving 600,000 dead and 1,200,000 injured: all these figures were based on calculations from the Spanish Civil War which had ended less than 6 months earlier. The actual civilian casualties in the whole of Great Britain from 6 years of war came to 295,000, of whom 60,000 were killed.

Because so many thousands of casualties were expected ,the current patients in all London hospitals were evacuated, and so were the prisoners in the next-door building of Wormwood Scrubs. In 1939 Sir Vernon Kell, head of MI5 – the national organization for internal security and counter-intelligence – found that the Security Service had outgrown its office space and so arranged a move to H.M. Prison, Wormwood Scrubs. On 23 August 1939, under the Emergency Orders Act, the 90 borstal trainees at Wormwood Scrubs were moved to Feltham so that A and D blocks of the prison were completely evacuated. For 3 nights the main doors were left open to allow the War Office to bring in equipment to furnish the cells as offices for the Staff of MI5. On 5 September the remaining prisoners were transferred elsewhere: the prison was not reopened until 1942 when 324 prisoners were received from Wandsworth, where bombing had been severe, but not all the accommodation was handed back until the end of the war.

The stream of smartly dressed, West End types turning up at the gates each morning for work naturally attracted a great deal of attention. Bus conductors on the No. 7 bus used to call out, 'All change for MI5' – when they reached the stop outside the prison. Many of the secretaries liked working at the Scrubs during that long, hot summer of 1940 because they could so easily spend their lunch-hour sunbathing on the grass at the back of the prison. There were several disadvantages; none of the cells had interior door-handles, doors accidentally shut would lock automatically, and there were no telephones.[44] The Signal Corps eventually supplied telephones to the more important offices but the cables were a serious hazard on the spiral staircases between cell floors. A massive card-index system containing information on the citizens of the country as far back as the Great War, and called the 'Registry' was guarded within the prison. Because of the fear that a bomb or fire would destroy this main weapon of home security, all data were photocopied and a second set stored at Blenheim Palace: 'convoys of Army trucks were escorted from the Scrubs, down the A40, through the village of Woodstock to the Palace. Police were located along the route in case of accidents although the utmost secrecy was demanded for the operation.' Inevitably, within days everyone in the village knew of the importance of Blenheim in spite of the fact that the Tenth Duke of Marlborough declined to move out of his own house: MI5 moved into rooms around him and erected huts in his grounds. Lady Kell, wife of the head of MI5 who was dismissed by Churchill in May 1940 having held the post since 1909, managed the canteen at Wormwood Scrubs. The prison staff were unable to take their new roles seriously, particularly when nothing much happened for 6 months after the declaration of war. The censorship department for all mail going overseas was housed next door to MI5 in the prison during 1940 and some aliens were detained in the Scrubs (and at Brixton and Holloway) as a form of preventive detection. For those working in the prison, life was probably quite exciting: many foreign agents (spies) were interrogated there and several 'turned' to become double agents for the British and from there to radio 'doctored' information.

Francis Fraser left the School to become Consultant in Medicine to, and later Director-General of, the Emergency Medical Service (E.M.S.), an organization devised by the Ministry of Health to cope with ordinary civilian sickness and for air-raid and Service casualties in the various parts of the country. The task was immense. In 1938 Britain there were two distinct systems of hospitals: the local authority hospitals and the voluntary hospitals. The two types differed in their origins, their evolution, their staffing, their finance and even their patients were different because they tended to care for different sections of the community. Each type was strongly rooted in its own tradition, and co-operation between them was the exception rather than the rule. Yet neither was responsible to any higher public authority to provide a comprehensive or balanced service. The total number of hospitals in England and Wales at that time was about 3000 (providing half-a-million beds) of which 1000 were voluntary: of the 750 voluntary general hospitals only 75 (including all the teaching hospitals) had more than 200 beds each and 500 had less than 100 beds.

In June 1938 the Emergency Medical Service was set up in preparation for war. The Civil Defence Act of 1939 made the Ministry of Health responsible for the treatment of all civilian casualties and the idea was to find 300,000 beds for them. This number was never achieved but many thousands of beds were put up, often in hutted accommodation in the grounds of hospitals outside London and the larger cities. Under the Act the Minister paid for structural improvements and new equipment. Many hospitials took advantage of this opportunity to re-equip and as a result, by the outbreak of war, 1000 new operating theatres had been installed, a civilian blood transfusion service developed, and an Emergency Public Health Laboratory Service started. Many doctors were recruited to full-time salaried posts and not allowed private practice.

It was only when a national survey was made from 1943 onwards[45] that the full picture was appreciated. It was depressing. Of the 2800 hospitals taken over by the N.H.S. in 1948, 45% had been built before 1891 and 24% before 1861 (at a time when the horse was the main means of transport): 'they stood where history and accident had placed them'.[46] The E.M.S. organized the hospital service into twelve regions (there are 14 regions in the 1984 N.H.S.) but London was divided into sectors, each sector widening outwards into the surrounding counties and based, in general, on one of the large teaching hospitals.

That 'something had to be done after the war' was generally agreed. The

N.H.S. Act of 1946 was based on the consensus that 'drastic changes were essential', which was all very well, but there was no agreement on the number of beds required for a given population or where they should be. The fact that a substantial proportion of the buildings were over 50 years old, many more than a century, meant that some could be modernized but others were hopeless and had to be rebuilt, yet nobody knew what a 'purpose-built hospital' should look like.

McMichael, as Reader, took over from Fraser the job of running the Department of Medicine 'for the duration', as it was called. Teaching and research continued in all departments but with depleted resources. The students attending included undergraduates from St Mary's Hospital who were provided with residential accommodation and completed their studies there, European refugees, and some nationals taking higher examinations – usually women, and men rejected for military service, or invalided out of the Services. 'Ward teaching can always be adapted to the intellectual level of the student under cross-examination: theatre lectures, however, cause difficulties owing to the gross inequality of training among the audience'.[47] The lectures evolved into tutorial discussions which held the interest of 'mixed junior and senior listeners'.

In the Hospital there was also a special unit for Czech soldiers and airmen, known as the Czech Hospital, which was visited by the President-in-exile and Madame Benes. The Hospital was hit by high explosive bombs and incendiaries on several occasions; the refectory where the opening ceremony had been held in May 1935 was destroyed and most windows were boarded up, but the Hospital, like many others, never had to close. The tuberculosis dispensary of Hammersmith Borough Council was destroyed by a bomb in January 1941 and moved to the Hospital where it has since remained, although with the different title of 'Chest Clinic'.

6

The Nationalization of Health Services and Federation of Postgraduate Institutes

In the Second World War the British people came of age because it was a people's war: they were all involved and they themselves wanted to win. Indeed the British, that is those of the Empire, Dominions and the United Kingdom, were the only people who fought continuously throughout both world wars from beginning to end. But, as already mentioned, the second war was vastly different from the first. 'The very spirit of the nation had changed. No one in 1945 wanted to go back to 1939. The majority were determined to go forward and were confident that they could do so'.[43] This was also the time when the Hammersmith changed from what others thought it should be to what those with more imagination and less tradition thought it could be. 'Imperial greatness was on the way out; the Welfare State was on the way in.' There was also mounting demand for a Welfare State as guarantee against any relapse to pre-war conditions.

THE BEVERIDGE PLAN

In 1941 Arthur Greenwood, deputy Leader of the Labour party, asked Sir William Beveridge to produce a plan for social welfare. The aspect of the report that caused most interest after the war was the proposal for a National Health Service to place everyone in an insurance scheme for medical treatment. The pre-war system had insured wage-earners, but not their wives and families, and had left salary-earners to make their own insurance arrangements. The detailed finances of the Report were hard to work out because wartime inflation was changing all wages and price levels, so Beveridge suggested that some benefits should increase by stages until their final value, perhaps 20 years after the war ended, but on the whole he set the pattern for all subsequent British thinking about Welfare. In 1942 the Beveridge Report was published, followed by a draft Bill (as a White Paper) in 1944.

Lord Beveridge's document was an extraordinarily naïve[48] and ignorant piece of work, which should have alarmed academics – certainly those at the Hammersmith – by its lack of sufficient facts discovered by enquiry. Admittedly, 40 years later the N.H.S. can be neither proud of, nor confident in, its own statistics, as the Korner Committee[49] of 1982 uncovered. The Beveridge Plan was founded on opinion, not research, and contained three major errors.

First, there did not exist a backlog of ill-health which was waiting to be cleared by a State Service to produce a healthy nation of reduced medical needs. On the contrary, new medical knowledge and techniques – many on view at Hammersmith at the time, and elsewhere, for anyone with eyes to see – produced new medical demands which seemed unlimited and occurred during the times of economic depression in the fifties and seventies.

Second, the plan depended on a well-financed and coherently organized national system of hospitals, which Francis Fraser among others had showed not to be so in Britain but the very reverse. Even in 1939, nearly all voluntary hospitals were heading for bankruptcy and the local authority hospitals were a drain on the rates. The Emergency Medical Service provided more beds but it did not create an organized system of equitable medical care, something that was still being debated in 1984.

Third, the plan required an equally well-equipped system of health centres to provide primary care from general practitioners, a situation that has only recently been accomplished. No wonder that within 5 years the cost of the N.H.S. had escalated in a way that alarmed those politicians who had been only too keen to take credit for its inception.

Understandably, as a result there was no new building, either of hospitals or of health centres, during the first 15 years of the N.H.S. Beveridge's plan was not researched but deduced from the supposed principles of social justice and social welfare: it was political ideology that was easier to accept than to argue about, at least until now. The union of health and social security by Richard Crossman in 1967 may have confirmed Virchow's comment of the previous century – 'Medicine is a social science and politics nothing else than medicine on a large scale' – but did nothing to solve the central problem of finance and expectations. Hammersmith recognized Virchow for his analysis of pathology, not for his sociology.

IMPLEMENTATION OF THE N.H.S.

Churchill's Caretaker Government of 1945 took the first step towards implementing Beveridge's recommendations by passing the Family Allowances Act. The main National Insurance Bill was made law in 1946, and the completion of the system of state financial provisions came with the National Assistance Act of 1948 which destroyed the last remnants of the Poor Law and ended workhouses. By this Act, all voluntary and municipal hospitals became vested in the Ministry, except a few which elected to remain outside the service. Previously, voluntary hospitals obtained some of their funds from legacies and public subscriptions – flag day appeals to the public were co-ordinated and King Edward's Hospital Fund and The British Hospital Association received and distributed the money according to proven needs – but much more came from payments, either direct or through a hospital savings association. Municipal hospitals, on the other hand, were rate-supported and all patients paid a proportion of full maintenance costs assessed on their financial circumstances. By the end of the war all hospitals were receiving large sums from the Ministry of Health, and the prospect of raising these amounts from voluntary sources at that time was remote.

Beveridge had worked out his plan for universal social security ('from the cradle to the grave') assuming the continued working of capitalism and, as Taylor in 1965 noted, 'finally rejected the Socialist doctrine of a social security provided by society. He took over the principle of a flat-rate contribution, which Lloyd George had unwillingly accepted in 1911 and so perpetuated, seemingly for ever, the retrograde principle of the poll-tax, against which Englishmen had revolted as long ago as 1381.' Strong words. Taylor also remarked that Beveridge got the job against his will: he wanted to plan the organization of labour but Bevan didn't like him and so wished him on to Greenwood. In 1943 the Churchill Coalition wartime government gave the report only faint blessing, but by 1945 it was part of the Labour election manifesto and on 5 July 1945 Labour won a landslide victory: Clement Attlee became Prime Minister and Aneurin Bevan Minister of Health.

The National Health Service (N.H.S.) set up under the Act of 1946 provided (virtually without charge to the individual) hospital and specialist services, general practitioner, ophthalmic, dental, maternity and child welfare, as well as the provision of drugs, medicines, dentures and spectacles. The cost was to be borne chiefly by the Exchequer out of general taxation. The Act was thus a major act of nationalization and turned voluntary hospitals into state-maintained ones, and the Health Service ended local authority control of other hospitals. Aneurin Bevan was in charge of the Bill. Teaching hospitals were excluded from the general organization and allowed separate Boards of Governors. To prevent the spread of private nursing homes Bevan agreed that single rooms and small wards in hospitals could be available to those prepared to pay extra for the privilege of privacy ('amenity' beds) and there was no bar to hospitals having their own private patients' block. General Practitioners would be independent contractors to the N.H.S., managed by local medical executive councils, and the whole of their remuneration would come from a capitation fee for each patient on their list. Specialists were paid a salary.

The N.H.S. was a major reform. Criticism after it began was mainly over its cost. In the first year over 5 million pairs of spectacles were issued and 187 million prescriptions for drugs written out. In 20 years it became the largest of the country's industries and the largest single item in the Budget after the defence forces. Later, Labour introduced charges for spectacles and dentures, and the Conservatives for prescriptions to limit costs, but by then medical advances, which were expensive and never envisaged originally, had taken over. Even in the first year the number of patients treated increased by 30%, but the total number of beds remained the same. The N.H.S. Act of 1946 came into force on 5 July 1948. Even though war was continuing, at first unsuccessfully, later with an end in sight, several other important changes were evolving. The Butler Education Act of 1944 was one milestone: it raised the school leaving age to 15 years and allowed part-time education until 18 years. Another Committee, under the Chairmanship of Sir William Goodenough,[50] was set up to examine education in Medical Schools and reported in 1944.

THE GOODENOUGH COMMITTEE AND THE POSTGRADUATE EDUCATION

The original Athlone Committe of 1921 had envisaged a Central University Hospital for London in close affiliation with various specialist hospitals, all providing postgraduate teaching. Before the war there was a central office at the London School of Hygiene and Tropical Medicine to which postgraduates could apply and be directed to the appropriate hospital of their needs. The Goodenough Report of 1944 supported the ideas put forward by representatives of the School and recommended that 'the British Postgraduate Medical School should be reconstituted as a federal organisation of which the Hammersmith (L.C.C.) Hospital and the teaching organisation with it would be one of the federated units. The other units would consist of a series of institutes, one in each of the principal special subjects, each of the institutes being based on a leading special hospital'. This was in fact tacit recognition that grafting the Postgraduate Medical School on to a municipal hospital in 1935 had been successful, and clearly was the way forward in the teaching of specialist subjects. In the event, things did not turn out that way and within 20 years the errors were easily identifiable.

The inter-departmental Committee on Medical Schools, chaired by Sir William Goodenough, reported to the Minister of Health (Rt Hon. Henry

Willink M.P.) and the Secretary of State for Scotland (Rt Hon. Thomas Johnston M.P.) in 1944, having had 50 meetings. The terms of reference, given in a letter of 7 April 1942, were: 'Having regard to the statement made by the Minister of Health in the House of Commons on 9 October 1941, indicating the Government's post-war hospital policy, to enquire into the organisation of Medical Schools, particularly in regard to facilities for clinical teaching and research, and to make recommendations'. It might be thought that conditions in the country were unlikely to lead to any worthwhile recommendations. In May 1940 the British Army had returned from Dunkirk and the Battle of Britain had lasted from July to September; in March 1941 the U.S.A. had passed the 'Lend-Lease' Act to allow Britain to continue the war; in June Hitler attacked Russia and appeared to be highly successful, and in December the Japanese attacked the U.S. fleet at Pearl Harbor. There appeared to be more important problems to consider than medical education, and some even doubted that London would remain a viable city.

Goodenough spoke of 'principles' of government and administration that had already been applied to undergraduate medical schools and should now also apply to the postgraduate hospitals – such as hospital, school, and university representation on governing bodies. One problem area which had been avoided by the Chamberlain Committee of 1930 was examined by the Goodenough Committee: what should be done about the various special hospitals in London? 'The special hospitals in London vary much in size, in equipment and in their staffing. Most of them have not organised schools at the present time and are not under any obligation to conform to university standards. They are not eligible for grants from the University and lack the money to enable them to develop postgraduate education on the lines they would like.' Goodenough recommended that:

- One special hospital in each major special subject should be brought up to university standards in staffing, accommodation and equipment.
- Each hospital will need to provide an adequate number of beds, and a suitable out-patient department.
- Each should have lecture rooms, library and reading rooms.
- Sufficient laboratory accommodation for the research work of both staff and postgraduate students should be provided.
- As each hospital or unit attained the desired standard to form its institute that institute should be federated to the British Postgraduate Medical School.
- Three hospitals (the Royal London Ophthalmic, the Hospital for Sick Children, and the National Hospital for Diseases of the Nervous System) already have 'recognised teachers of the University' on their staff and should be first to federate.

The Goodenough Report referred to the Medical School as the 'Hammersmith Postgraduate Institute' and the term 'British Postgraduate Medical School' was used to refer to the proposed federal organization. The central office was to be in the centre of London near to the University and not attached to any of the institutes. As a result, the Postgraduate Medical Federation was established by Royal Charter on 31 March 1947. By a supplementary Charter the name of the British Postgraduate Medical School was changed to the 'Postgraduate Medical School of London'. An Academic Board was established by the Committee of Management of the School (which replaced the Governing Body of the School constituted by the original charter) to replace the School Council. The Academic Board was to consist of:

- all members of the staff who were University Professors,
- the Dean of the School,
- two representatives of the Readers and other whole-time members of the staff of the School of the status of Lecturers, to be appointed annually by the Board, and
- two representatives of the part-time permanent staff of the School to be appointed annually by the Board.

The Academic Board could appoint representatives to the Committee of Management, to the Central Academic Council of the Federation, to the Board of Advisers for the appointment of Professors and Readers, to the Senate for 'recognition' of teachers in the School.

So it came to pass that separate Institutes were created within the Federation but more loosely linked than Goodenough wished: for Psychiatry, Child Health, Laryngology and Otology, Diseases of the Chest, Orthopaedics, Dermatology, Cardiology, Urology, Dental Surgery, Ophthalmology, Neurology, Obstetrics and Gynaecology. There is little doubt that by agreeing to become part of the Federation – on the grounds that individual Institutes would not grow and could not survive alone without a general hospital – the Hammersmith made a great sacrifice, at a time when it could ill afford this gesture, and was bitterly to regret its philanthropy; it ceased to be an independent School within the University of London and in the Robbins Committee Report[51] of July 1964, Hammersmith was not even mentioned by name, only the Federation, although all the London undergraduate hospitals were.

Almost the only good thing for Hammersmith to come out of the Goodenough Report was that the School needed 'reorganisation, increase in staff and extensive additions to the accommodation . . . the urgent requirements include lecture theatres, demonstration rooms and laboratories of various kinds in both hospital and school buildings, staff rooms, and reasonable social amenities for staff and students, an enlarged library and museum, and an animal house of adequate size. The Out-patient accommodation of the hospital is too small. In short what the teaching departments at

Hammersmith Hospital need is the staff and accommodation which were originally proposed, and which no doubt they would have received but for the financial crisis of 1931.' None of these items materialized within the next 10 years, and some are still requirements at the time of writing in 1984. To compound the confusion, part of the Institute of Child Health remained at Hammersmith (the main part being in Queen Square) as did part of the Institute of Obstetrics and Gynaecology (the remainder being at Queen Charlotte's Hospital and Chelsea Hospital for Women).

The recommendations of the Goodenough Committee were based on pre-war practices and on the continuation of a sizeable private practice section in the country. The Committee could not have been expected to see the dramatic new developments in medicine and their economic, social and managerial effects on patients in hospital. Besides, wartime was hardly the right time to review medical education because war experience and penicillin were to change the outlook of doctors and patients radically and permanently. Even so a surprising number of recommendations were adopted. For the Hammersmith, the most important was the concept of a Federation for Postgraduate Hospitals.

7
Peacetime Hammersmith

As the transition from war to peace accelerated, the number of doctors at the Hammersmith increased tenfold. Service doctors, on demobilization, were offered posts for 6 months equivalent to Registrar status and pay in the specialty they had been studying before the war as part of their re-education to civilian life and in lieu of a 'gratuity' for service to their country. In 1945 there was no nostalgia for the 'good old days': all wanted fuller social justice, greater security and peace, and a lessening of class differences.[52] Hammersmith wanted a meritocracy and it says much for morale that, in the midst of all the confusion and relocation, School staff were able to continue their work and expand into new fields. The place filled up with men of wider experience and an impatience with the stuffier aspects of tradition: many were single-minded and ruthless in their pursuit of academic success. Apart from those attending special courses, 913 students enrolled in 1945 and 674 in 1946. By 1950 the total was down to 438, but more than half came from overseas: this ratio, in an average total of 420–480, was to remain fairly constant for the next 5 years, and about half spent 6 months or more at the School.

In 1946 the School Governing Body appointed a committee to consider moving the School to a more central site in London – nearer to the great libraries, other institutes in the Federation, and the University – even if the existing and very inadequate transport facilities were improved, which seemed unlikely if not impossible. The committee never reported, but a School omnibus to and from White City station (a shuttle service for students) was run in 1947. Restrictions on petrol rationing reduced the extent of the service and eventually the authorities vetoed the 'use of the van for the convenience of doctors attending as students': the van was retained for general duties, replaced today by a School car.

STAFF CHANGES

There were changes in senior consultant staff. Professor Grey Turner had remained in post during the war, until the age of 69, and still operated although severely crippled by rheumatoid arthritis, to be succeeded by Ian Aird, a Lieutenant-Colonel and Surgical Specialist of wartime and at 41[53] the youngest Professor in the University. Grey Turner believed and preached that an academic surgeon should experiment and push ahead into the unknown for the benefit of patients, for no one else can break new ground without questionable motives. Aird, his successor, a Scot with the gift of words and mellifluous phrases, wrote of him: 'As first occupant of the chair of a new university venture, Grey Turner was a perfect choice for he brought to it his personal fame as one of the leaders of British Surgery, an established reputation as a teacher, a gift of authority, high manual dexterity, and surgical ingenuity and courage tempered, as not always, by ruthless self-criticism and unfailing common sense. His successes in resection of the oesophagus and in the treatment of malignant disease of the bladder would themselves have been sufficient to justify his tenure of the postgraduate chair. He established by his practice of it, the principle that one of the duties of the whole-time academic surgeon is to undertake the early stages of development of surgical operations of great magnitude and risk, and to repeat them in spite of early disappointment, if they are demanded by extensive disease, proved possible by animal experiment, justified by physiology, and sanctioned by humanity. Grey Turner's success in two unhappy fields of malignant disease is proof of the propriety of this argument, in his own hands at least.'

Professor Sir Francis Fraser left in 1946 to become the first Director of the British Postgraduate Medical Federation, at the Headquarters in Guildford Street, to be succeeded by John McMichael[54] as Professor of Medicine. Professor James Young retired in 1948 to be succeeded by John McClure Browne as Professor of Obstetrics and Gynaecology. Professor Henry Dible did not retire until 1954 when Vic Harrison took his post as Professor of Morbid Anatomy, but by then the Department of Pathology had virtually divided into several autonomous departments, each with its own professor, the most senior acting as Chairman of the Division, and none of the professors holding established rank in the University (which was soon rectified).

Sir Thomas Carey Evans retired as Medical Superintendent in 1945 to be succeeded by Dr H. G. Wimbush. In the same year Miss G. M. Godden became the Matron when Miss Campbell was promoted to County Hall.

As a teaching hospital, the Hammersmith had its own Board of Governors, responsible direct to the Minister of Health. The Minister had decided, for convenience of administration, that the West London Hospital and St Mark's Hospital for Diseases of the Rectum should be linked to Hammersmith and the same governing body control all three. The first Chairman of the Board was Mr Somerville Hastings M.S., F.R.C.S., M.P., who had been Chairman of the Hospitals and Medical Services Committee of the L.C.C. William Milton, previously steward of the Hospital, was appointed secretary to the Board (and was to be a prime mover in what came to be known as 'The 1951 Agreement').

THE 1951 AGREEMENT

The N.H.S. Act of 1946 seemed to be working well in the years after its implementation on 5 July 1948, but there were several problem areas which had been neglected or debarred from full discussion: for instance the place of full-time academic university staff in the organization had never been defined. The discussions which led to the '1951 Agreement' took place during 1949 to 1951, in letters exchanged between the Ministry of Health, the Principal of the University of London, the British Postgraduate Medical Federation, the School, and with the Board of Governors of Hammersmith Hospital late in 1950, the main provisions are summarized in the letter reproduced here:

> Ministry of Health,
> Whitehall SW1.
> REF; 94/3/3
> 23 January 1951
> I am glad to say that we have now got general agreement about the clinical staff at the Hammersmith Hospital (about which you last wrote to Mr. Pater on 22 December 1950).
>
> The Agreement as finally reached is as follows:
>
> (a) The Medical Superintendent, the staff of the Radiodiagnostic and Radiotherapy Departments, the Medical Officers in the chest clinics and the two Senior Dental Officers will be paid by the Board of Governors.
>
> (b) All other members of the medical staff of Hammersmith Hospital, whether full-time or part-time, who are consultants or Senior Hospital Medical Officers, will be paid by the School out of University funds and will hold honorary contracts only with the Board of Governors. (Distinction awards will, of course, be payable by the Board of Governors in the ordinary way, subject to the last paragraph of this letter.)
>
> (c) The Board of Governors will not make any payment to the School towards the cost of staff paid by the School, except on an agreed basis for services rendered by the Department of Pathology as a Department.
>
> I understand that the School will now be asking for honorary contracts for the clinical teachers referred to in (b) and there is, of course, no reason why these contracts should not be allowed.
>
> As to distinction awards for the staff in (b) who are eligible for such

awards, I am afraid the position at the moment still remains that the general question of the payment of such awards to clinical teachers who hold honorary contracts with a Hospital Board is under review and for the time being we have told all Boards not to pay awards to such staff, but simply to inform the Minister of the names of the staff concerned (see paragraph 11(1) (a) 1(ii) of the official letter which was sent to all Boards on 18 September 1950, under reference 94112/4/1. As soon as we have got the position straightened out we shall, of course, be sending a further communication to all Boards.

Yours sincerely (Signed) A S Marre.

William Milton Esq. Secretary to the Board of Governors Hammersmith Hospital.

This '1951 Agreement', hailed as a reasonable and just compromise for the future of the Hammersmith at the time, was to become restrictive and unyielding to progress within a decade. In effect the agreement stated that all senior (consultant) staff at the School would be employees of the University and would run clinical services in the Hospital: the N.H.S. would supply the necessary junior staff for these consultants. The central fault in the scheme was not spotted at the time: the School staff failed to realize that they could not increase the number of Lecturers (Consultants in the N.H.S.) indiscriminately and expect junior staff to be supplied and paid for automatically.

SOCIAL AND HOSPITAL CHANGES

The years 1945 to 1951 were a time of social revolution and of depression too. In 1947 there had been a dollar crisis in the U.S.A., a severe winter with bread and potatoes rationed for the first time in the U.K., and a fuel crisis. In 1947 the Marshall Plan for relief in Europe was initiated – the aluminium U.S. Army Quonset hut erected between C and D blocks at the front of the hospital site, to house the Blood Transfusion Research Unit in 1951, was one donation – and Sir Francis Fraser became Vice-Chancellor of the University. In July 1950 the U.S.A. was involved in the war in Korea, and by October there was a financial crisis in Britain so that patients were required to contribute 50% of the cost of their N.H.S. spectacles – by Hugh Gaitskell who had succeeded Stafford Cripps as Chancellor of the Exchequer. The feeling that life was getting better in the country was stimulated by Herbert Morrison's 'Festival of Britain' in 1951, although critics have since derided its importance and logic: there was no logic, simply a communal feeling to smile in adversity. In February of the next year King George VI died and the 'Festival' spirit was revived by the coronation of Queen Elizabeth II in 1953.

Hammersmith in 1955 had changed considerably from the place it had been in 1935. Nursing staff had increased to nearly 600 – the new Nurses Home,

Hammersmith House built in 1938, was now too small to accommodate all (it was built for 346) – the training school had an annual intake of 140 nurses from 30 countries. A hospital staff restaurant, rebuilt in 1951 having been destroyed by a bomb during the war, was opened by the Rt Hon. Herbert Morrison M.P., the then Secretary of State for Foreign Affairs, who in earlier years had been associated with the Hospital. The restaurant was on two floors, providing a waitress service on the ground floor and a cafeteria on the upper floor, seating 450, and this then released the original dining room in Hammersmith House for recreation. The Premature Baby Unit, opened in 1947, on the ground floor ward of F block, had developed into an important part of paediatrics: there were 20 cots and on the floor above five bedrooms for nursing mothers. Most of the babies admitted to the unit had been born in the Maternity Wards of the Hammersmith, but an increasing number came from other hospitals as its value became recognized: in 7 years the mortality of premature babies admitted had fallen from 20% to 13% and in 1955 the smallest baby to survive weighed only 1 lb 13 oz at birth. The Sister in charge, Miss Castle, retired in 1982 after 30 years service, and the total number of babies that she had managed was estimated to be well over 5000. Student Nurses attended the unit from Great Ormond Street Hospital (the Institute of Child Health) as did pupil midwives from Hammersmith.

In 1951 the Board of Governors had negotiated for King Edward's Hospital Fund to purchase a convalescent home (St Helena's Recovery Home in Cricklewood) and lease it to the Board. It had 22 beds but was never fully occupied after about 1960 and so was relinquished in 1974. In 1955 a new operating theatre was constructed off the North Corridor of the hospital, F Theatre, later to be converted to the more productive renal dialysis unit. The 1952 plan to create four new operating theatres on the top of D block, above the two originally built before the war by the London County Council (the original theatres were then to be converted to a ward (D9) for cardiac surgery), was not implemented until 1958.

Tuberculosis was still a serious and common disease. When the Hammersmith Borough Chest Clinic had been bombed, temporary accommodation was provided in the Hospital, but when the N.H.S. was inaugurated in 1948 responsibility for the clinic devolved upon the Board of Governors. The number of patients seen and treated had increased – and were to remain high, as tuberculosis gave way to lung cancer and bronchitis in the next 20 years – so that the clinic had to be moved to larger premises on the ground floor of I block, and two wards of 27 beds above the clinic were set aside for patients with tuberculosis, as were additional beds at St Charles Hospital (and staffed by Hammersmith nurses). The mortality from pulmonary tuberculosis in England and Wales fell from nearly 20,000 in 1949 to less than 4000 in 1959: mass miniature radiography discovered an average of 3.7 cases per thousand population in 1949 and only 1.9 in 1958.

The Board built an extension to the north side of B block as a special unit of eight beds and a laboratory for the investigation of metabolic disorders in 1950 and in 1952 added a 'clinic room' (for demonstration and teaching on individual patients) as a vertical extension at the entrance to B block medical wards. A central sterile syringe and needle supply service was set up in 1954 in a spare hut behind B block, but was overtaken by the marketing of disposables in 1960 and abandoned: the premises were converted for a central sterile supply of standardized dressings.

After the Medical Research Council's Radiotherapeutic Unit came to Hammersmith in 1942 the number of patients treated from that and the surrounding hospitals had steadily increased: in 1954 the M.R.C. had erected a new building to house a linear accelerator at one end and a cyclotron at the other. Above were three floors of laboratories. The Hospital Board paid for and added an extra floor for use by the School as a research laboratory for research into isotopes in the treatment of disease.

THE GUILLEBAUD COMMITTEE

When the Conservative Party came to power in 1951 they were committed to making the National Health Service more 'efficient' (both parties still promised this in the eighties). So, in April 1953 Iain Macleod, the new Minister of Health, announced that an independent enquiry would be chaired by Mr Claude Guillebaud,[55] a Cambridge economist, 'to determine how increasing costs could be avoided while maintaining the service and to make recommendations on how the service could be modified'. For the next 30 years this was to be the holy grail for which all political parties searched. No one would admit that medicine might be changing, that modern medicine could be costly, that free-for-all medicine might be impracticable.[56] Labour feared that this was a subversive attempt to reduce the service and Conservatives expected news of extravagant and wasteful practices. The Committee's report in 1956 pleased neither party. It showed that increased costs were due to increase in prices (inflation) and increased number of patients using the service (a larger population receiving more treatment); it stated that the rate of expenditure on the N.H.S. was too low! Worse still it found that 'many of the hospital buildings were inadequate at the time of inception of the National Health Service and many were badly sited'. The Guillebaud Committee recommended that the Government should treble the capital investment in hospitals and found no evidence of extravagance in the National Health Service. In fact, no new hospitals of any appreciable size were built in Britain in the period 1948 to 1960, in spite of the recommendation. In the U.S.A. during this same period 3000–4000 new hospitals were completed to provide 135,000 new beds! (More than half had fewer than 50 beds, 20% had 50–90 beds and the remaining 30% had 100 beds or more: it should be noted that new private hospitals built in the U.K. in the 1980s were generally small and essentially for acute services.)

But the amount of new building on the Hammersmith site was negligible when compared with that required, and when no new hospital materialized the Hammersmith solution was huts.

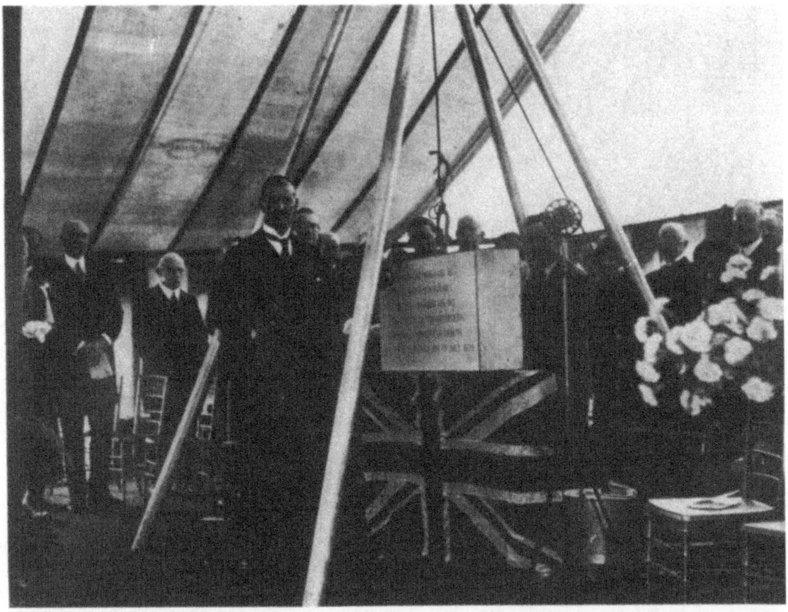

Figure 1 11 July 1933. Neville Chamberlain, Chancellor of the Exchequer, lays the foundation stone of the Postgraduate Medical School

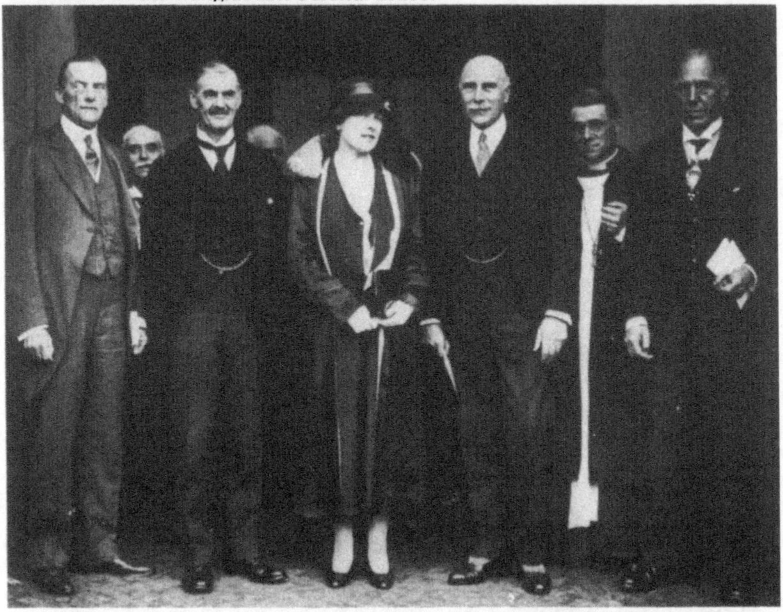

Figure 2 11 July 1933. At the foundation ceremony. Left to right: Sir Austen Chamberlain (Chairman of the Governing Body), Neville Chamberlain, Countess Athlone, Earl Athlone (Chancellor of the University), Bishop of Kensington, Mayor of the Borough of Hammersmith. Professor Gask (Chairman of the School Council) is at the back between the Chamberlains

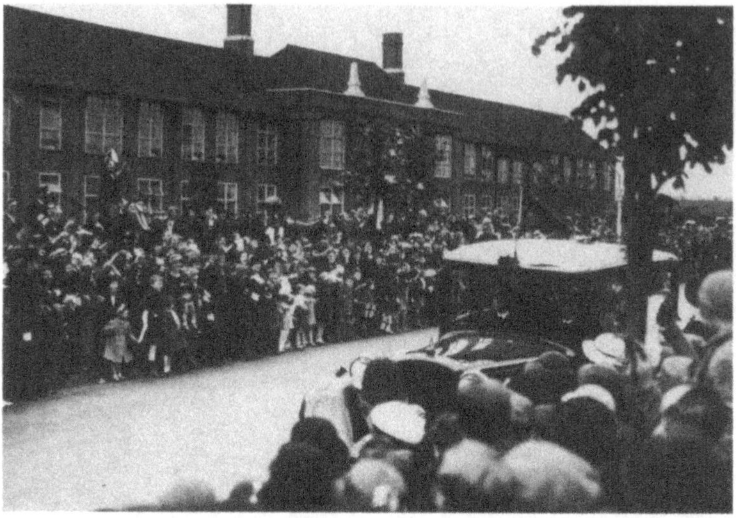

Figure 3 13 May 1935. The Royal car (a Daimler, of course) passing St Clement Danes School before turning into the Hospital grounds

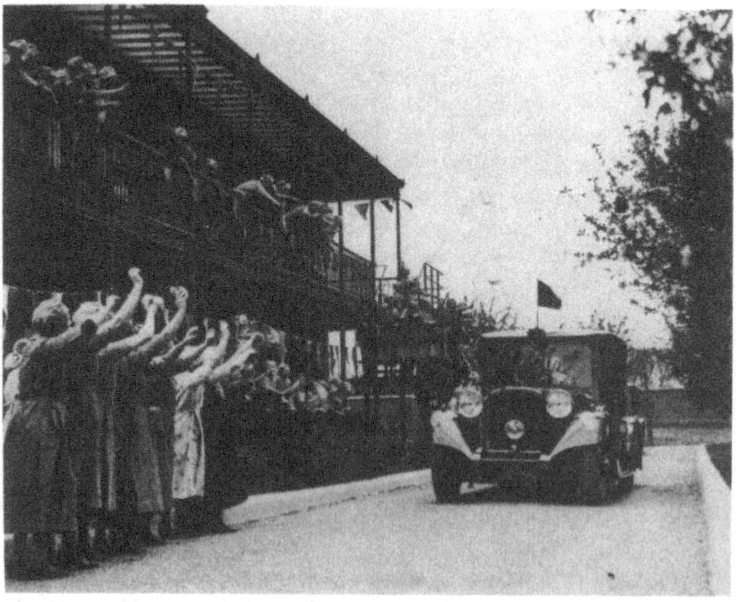

Figure 4 13 May 1935, Ward nurses cheer the Royal car. Note the open balconies, and nurses' uniforms, especially the caps

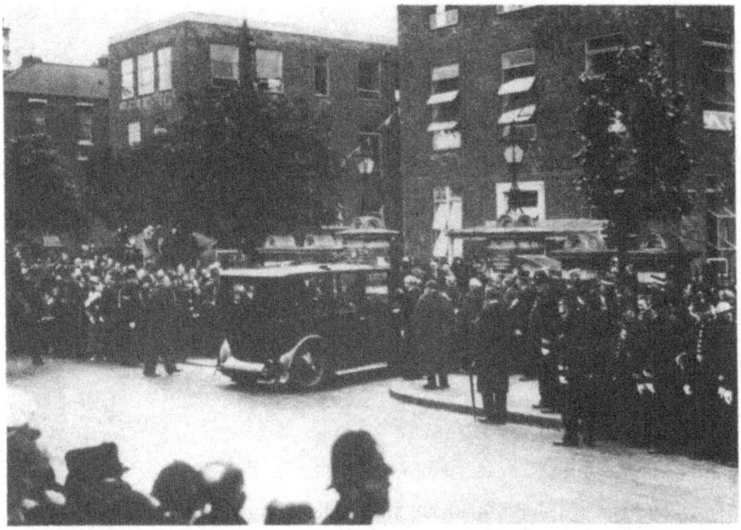

Figure 5 13 May 1935. The Royal car enters the School gate (the East gate) and is welcomed by the Mayor of Hammersmith Borough with the Town Clerk standing behind him

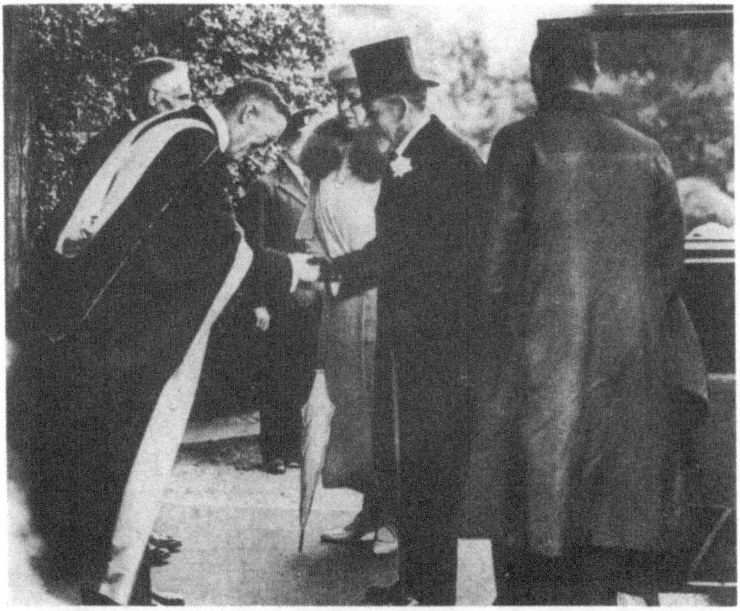

Figure 6 13 May 1935. King George V and Queen Mary are greeted by Professor Filon, Vice-Chancellor of the University

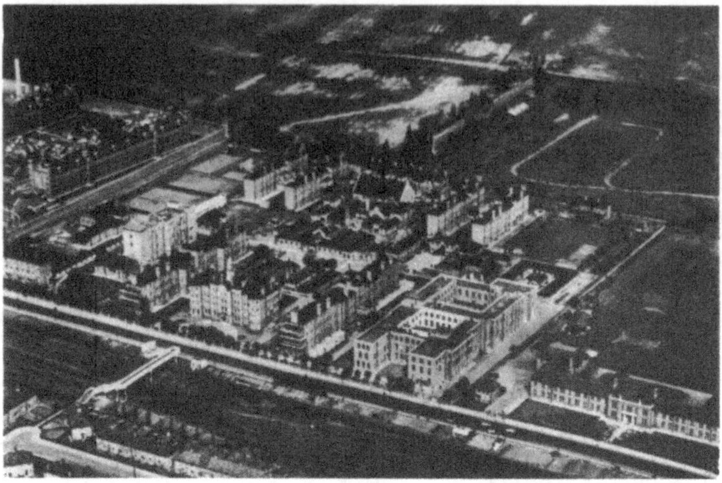

Figure 7 *c*. 1936. The British Postgraduate Medical School and Hammersmith Hospital, aerial view. Note, centre, the high-roofed refectory where the opening ceremony was held in 1935, bombed in 1942. Above, the Army recruiting huts have been removed but the rifle range and the loop road remain. Left, Wormwood Scrubs Prison. Right of main site, the Medical School. Right of photo, St Clement Danes School and playing fields. This photograph was issued as a postcard for overseas students to buy and send home

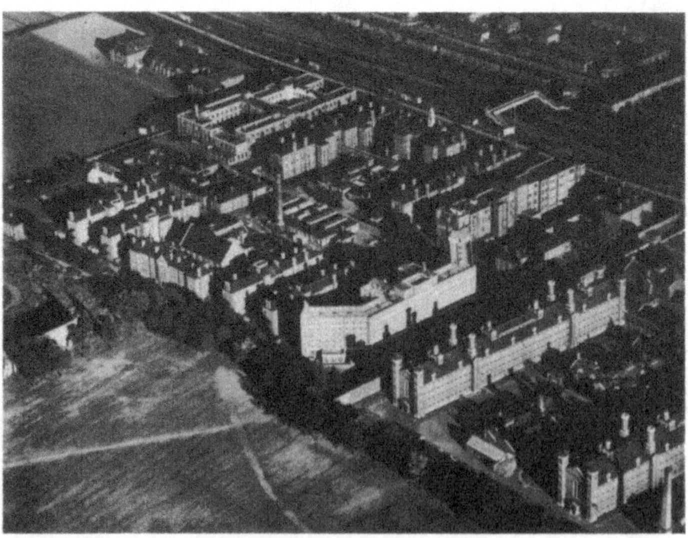

Figure 8 *c*. 1938. Aerial view of the Hospital and School. Note, bottom right, prison buildings and (centre) the new Nurses' Home

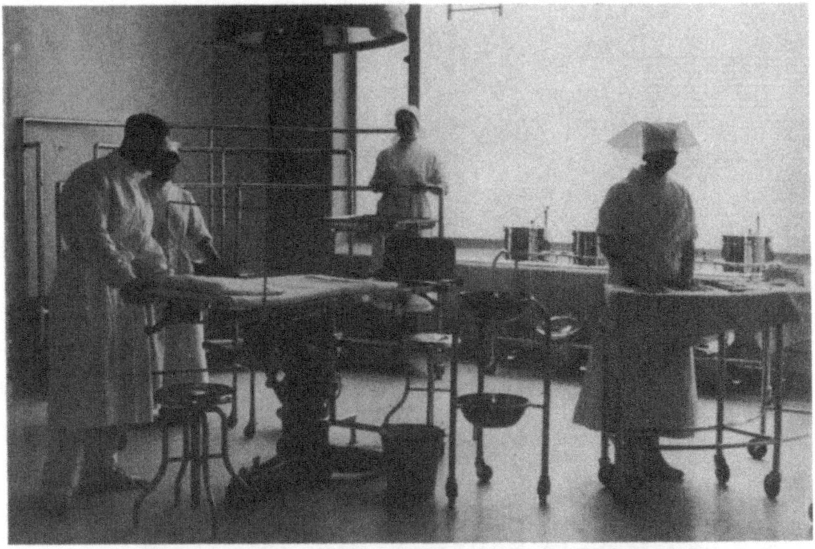

Figure 9 *c.* 1936. The new operating theatre on the top of D block. Note the rails and stands for visiting surgeons to watch operations. Theatre staff wore white gowns: green was introduced after the war

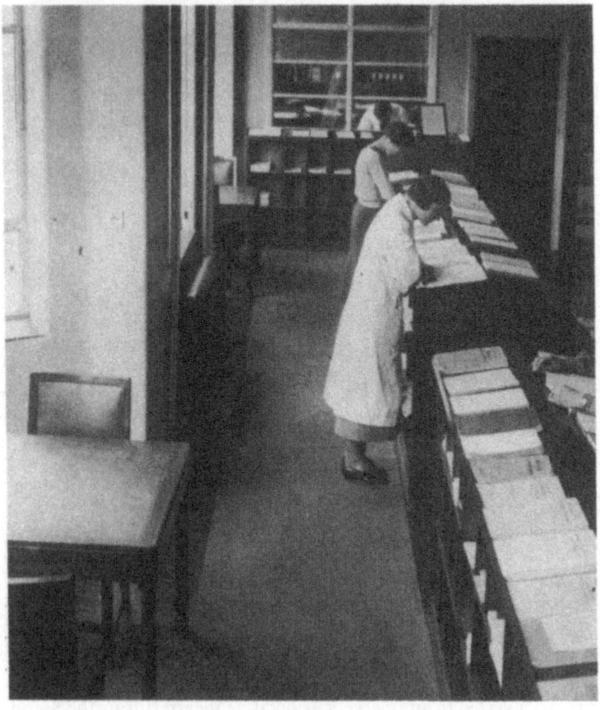

Figure 10 *c.* 1936. The School library in L block, looking towards the issue desk and office

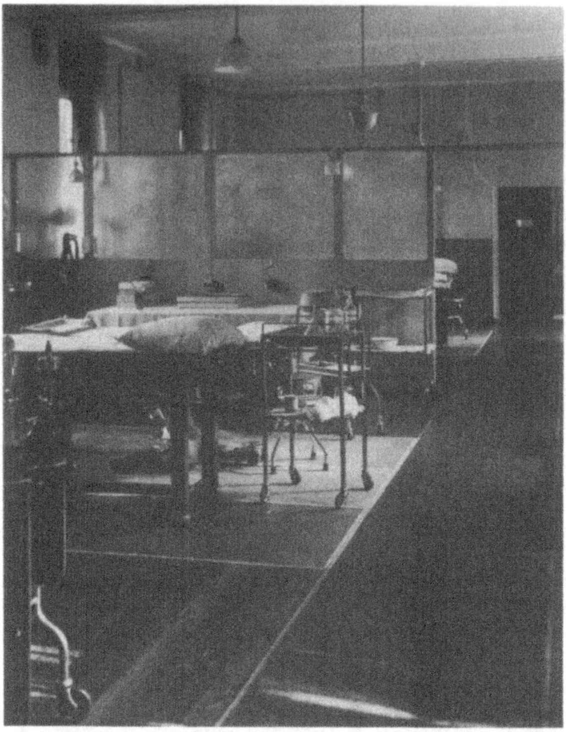

Figure 11 *c.* 1940. Ward C2 converted to an anaesthetic room (operating theatre seen beyond) during wartime. Note floor linoleum limited to main walk-ways

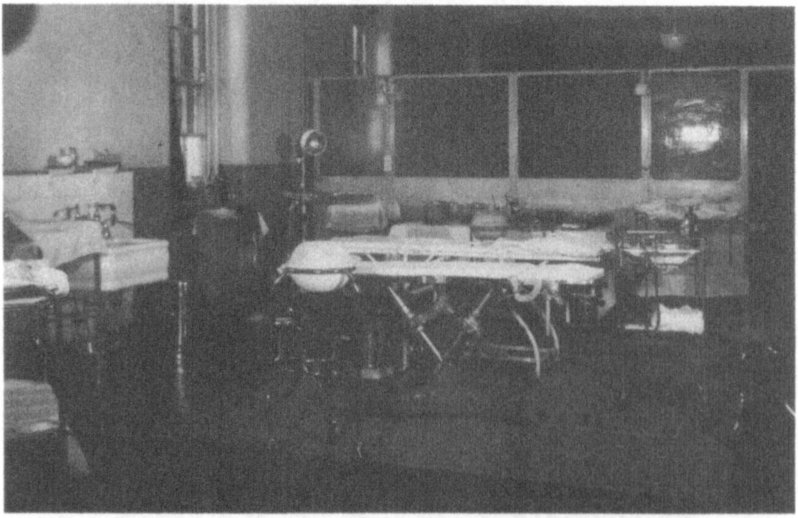

Figure 12 Ward C2 converted to an emergency operating theatre during the Second World War, about 1940

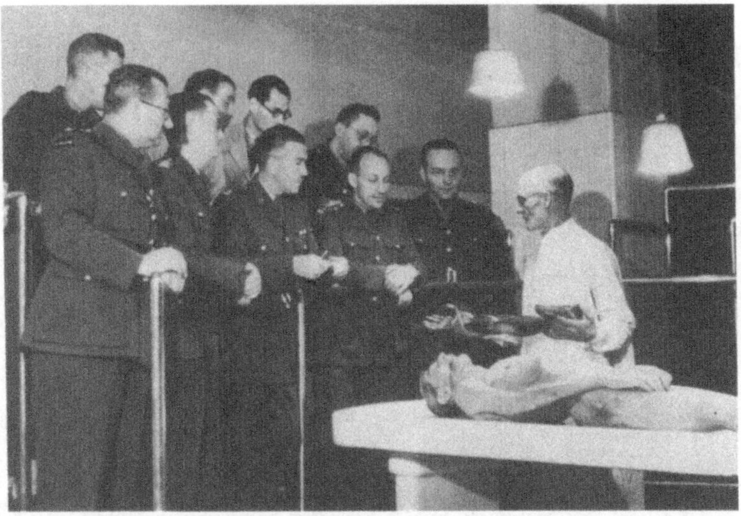

Figure 13 *c*. 1942. Canadian Army doctors attending a post-mortem demonstration. Note shoulder flashes

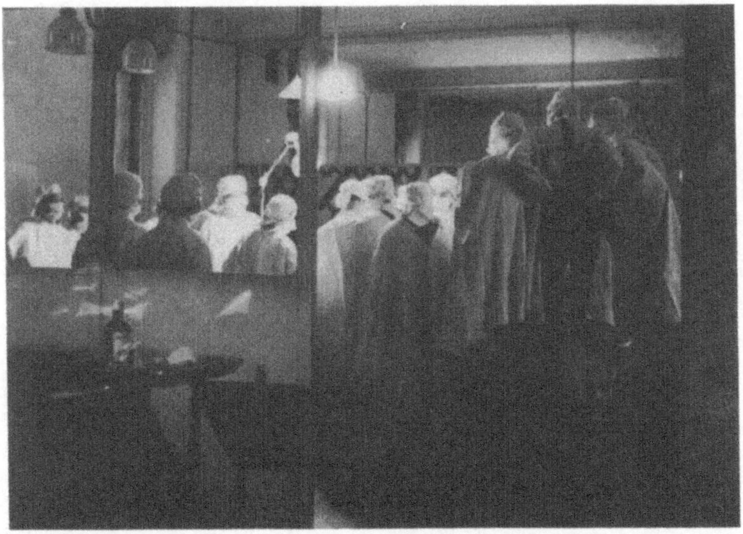

Figure 14 Visiting doctors watching an operation in the emergency theatre in a modified ground-floor ward

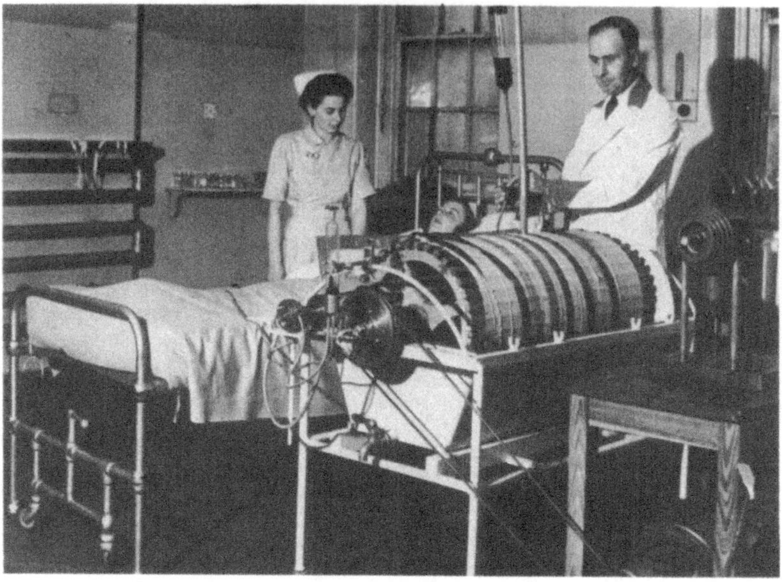

Figure 15 *c.* 1947. The Kolff artificial kidney machine, the first in the world: designed and built in Holland during the German Occupation

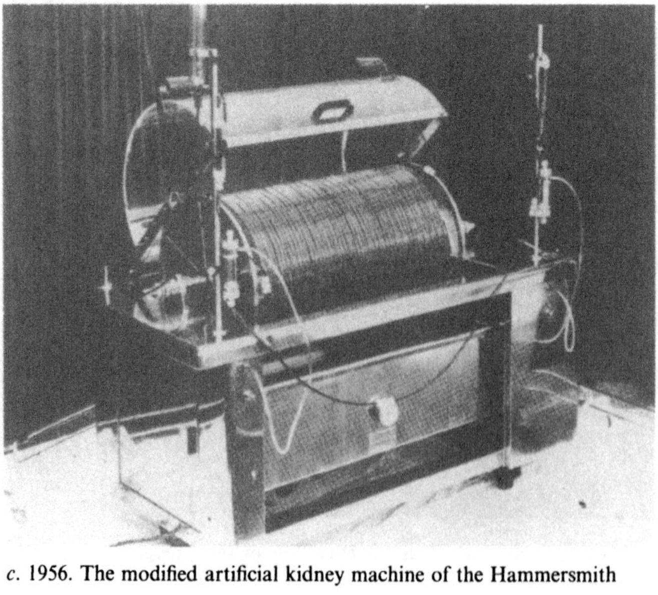

Figure 16 *c.* 1956. The modified artificial kidney machine of the Hammersmith

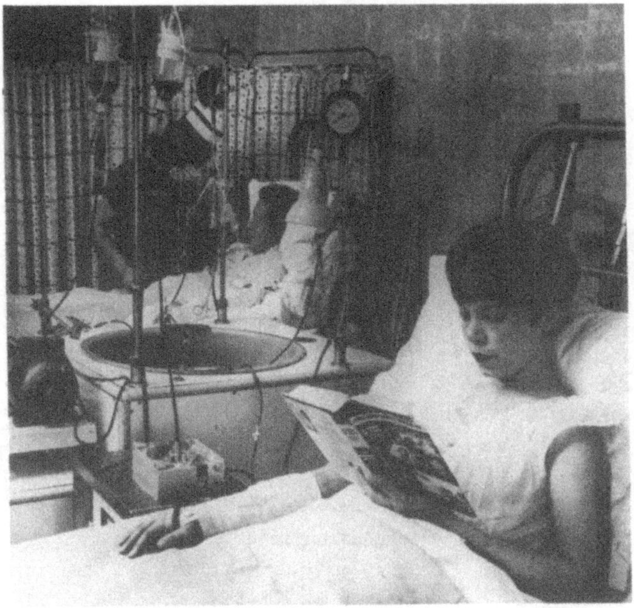

Figure 17 *c*. 1967. Renal dialysis in a special ward unit

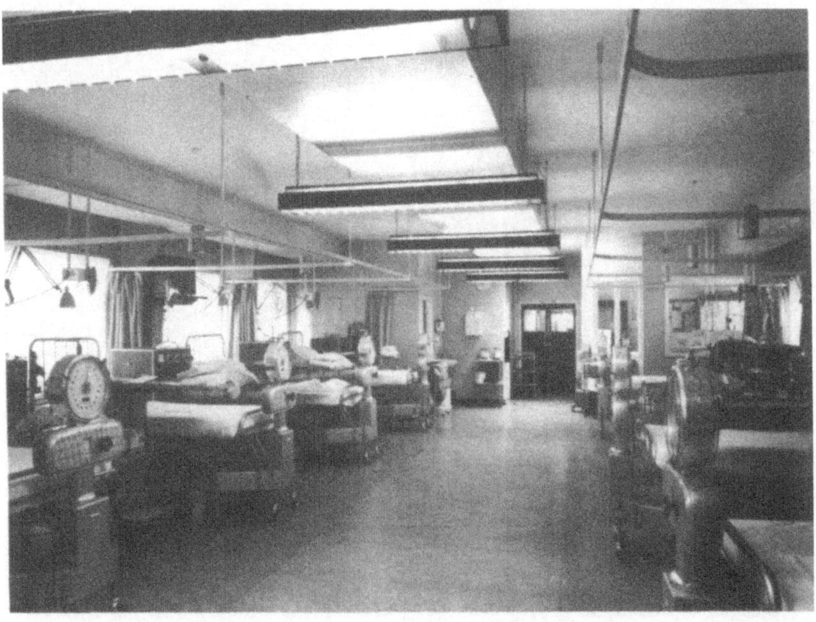

Figure 18 *c*. 1967. The Renal Dialysis ward of eight machines, used for day and night shifts (16 patients daily). Note calibrated scales of bed-weighing machines at the foot of each bed

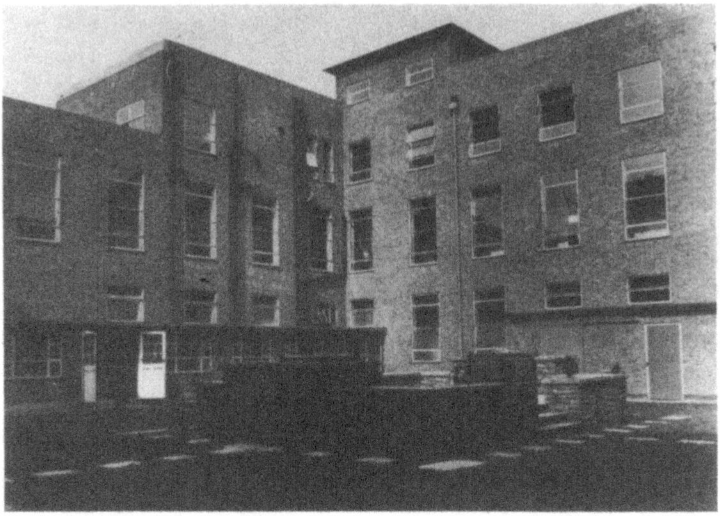

Figure 19 *c*. 1956. The Medical School quadrangle and Dean's garden

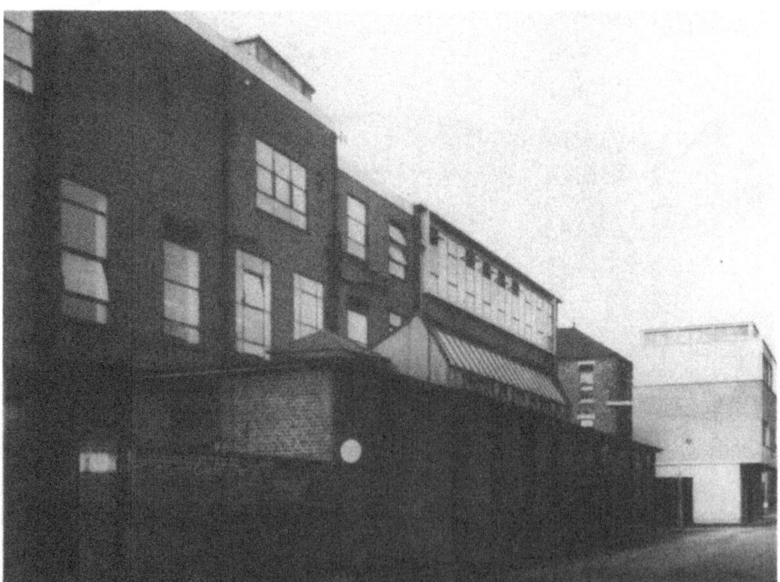

Figure 20 *c*. 1956. The back of the Medical School (mortuary and path. labs, with north-facing windows). To the right of the picture is the Metabolic Unit, erected by the Hospital in 1955

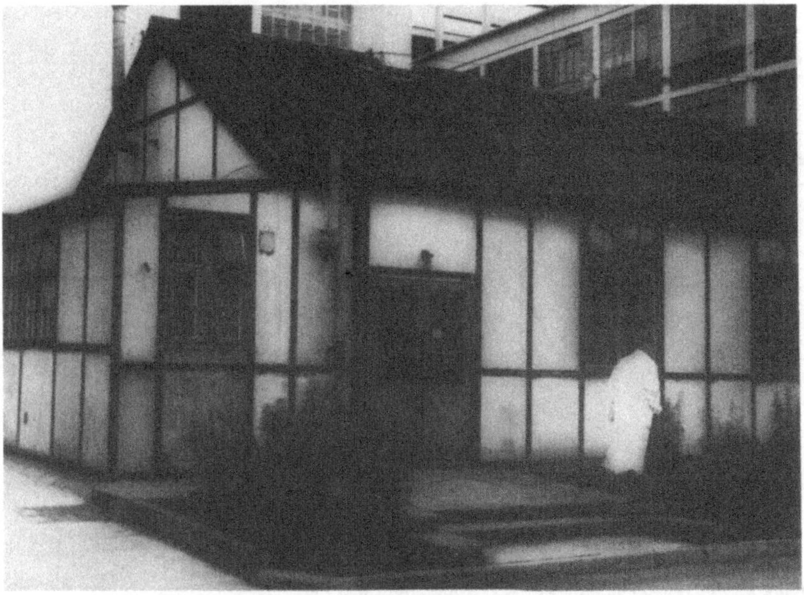

Figure 21 *c.* 1956. The School refectory hut (the doctors' mess): originally it had been used by Sir Robert Jones for making artificial limbs in 1917. Note above, the M.R.C. Cyclotron Building, the fourth floor just visible with elaborate gantries, which was completed in time for the Hospital Jubilee in 1955

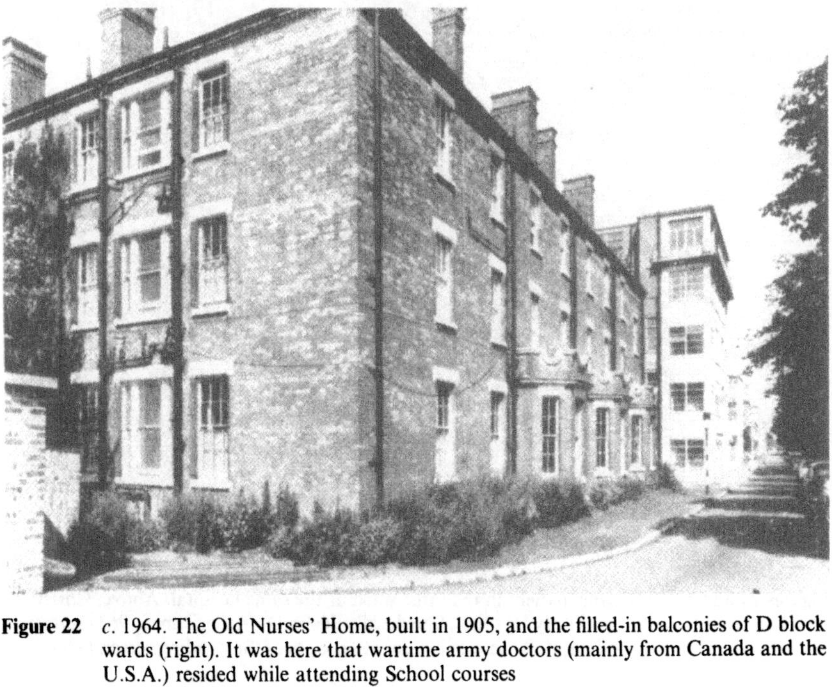

Figure 22 *c.* 1964. The Old Nurses' Home, built in 1905, and the filled-in balconies of D block wards (right). It was here that wartime army doctors (mainly from Canada and the U.S.A.) resided while attending School courses

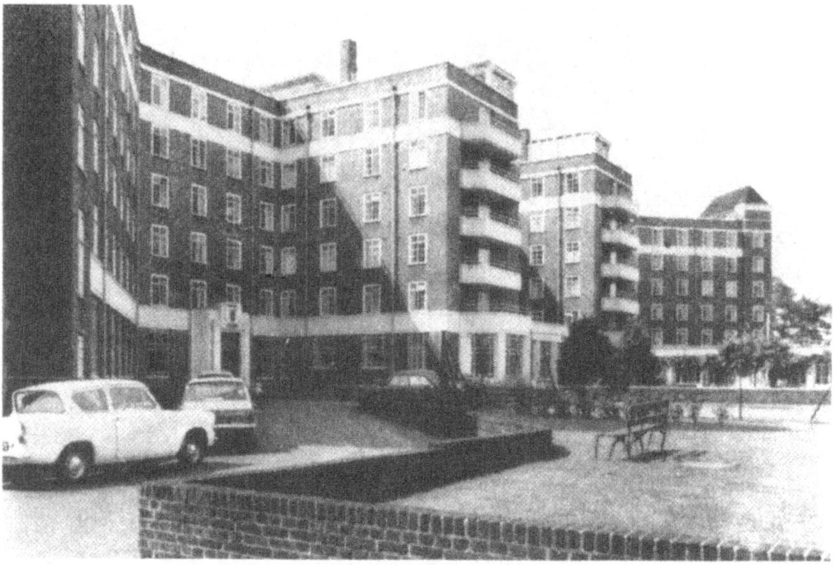

Figure 23 *c.* 1964. The New Nurses' Home, built in 1938

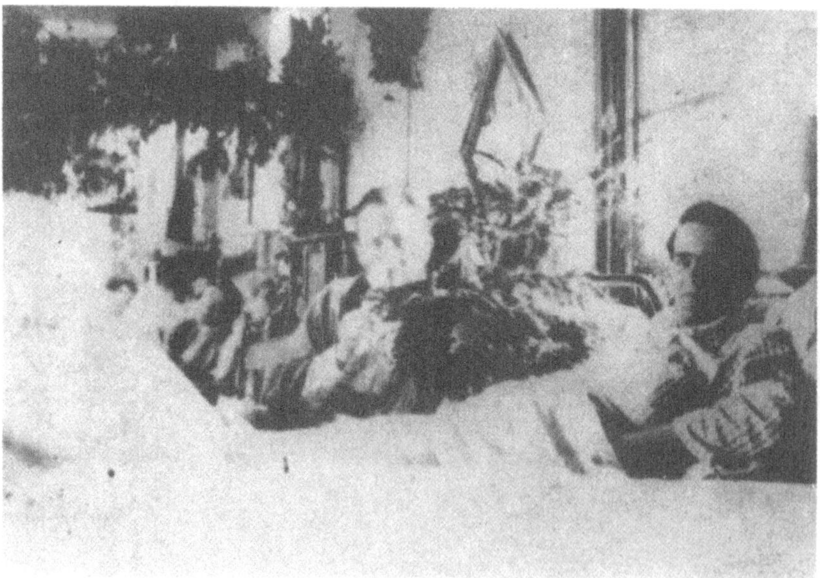

Figures 24 and 25 The same patient in the same ward of the same hospital. Above, Christmas 1917 (Military Hospital, Shepherd's Bush). Over, Christmas 1963 (Hammersmith Hospital): note crib painted on glass of the dividing screen behind the bed

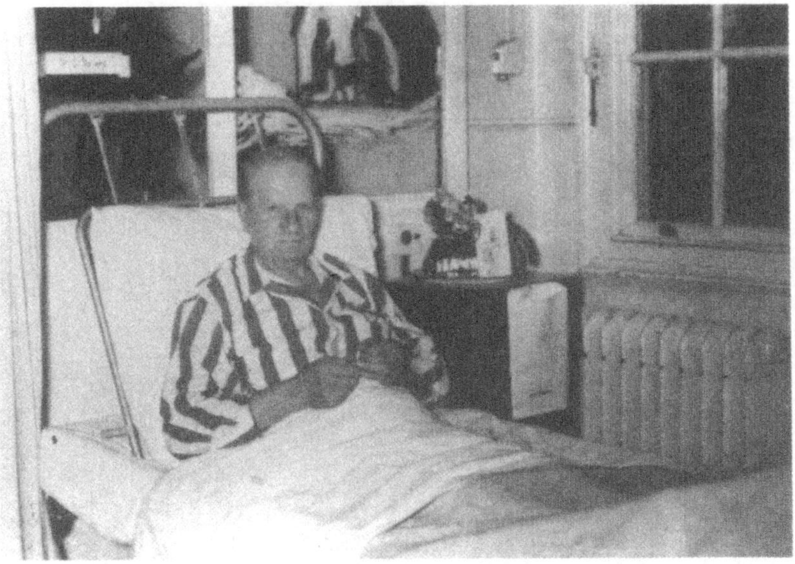

Figure 25

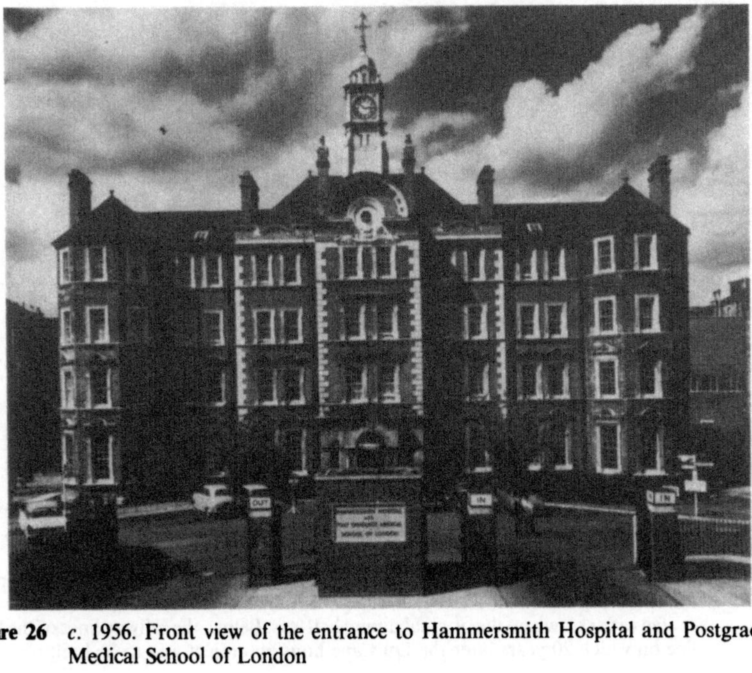

Figure 26 *c*. 1956. Front view of the entrance to Hammersmith Hospital and Postgraduate Medical School of London

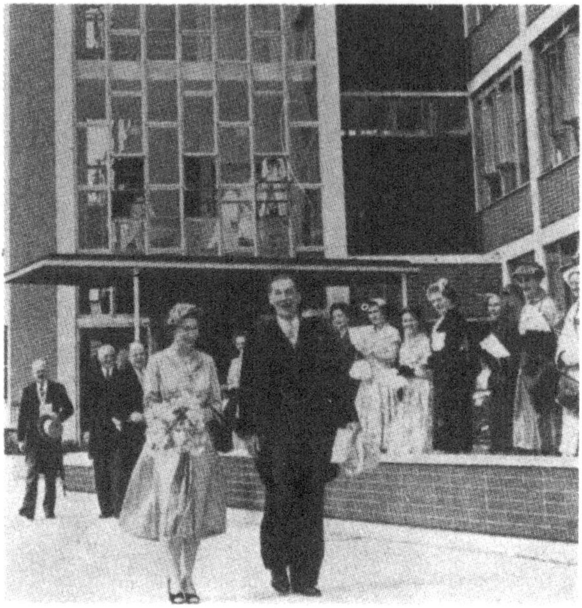

Figure 27 6 June 1955. H.M. Queen Elizabeth leaving the Cyclotron Building (completed in October 1954) on the occasion of the Golden Jubilee of Hammersmith Hospital, accompanied by Sir Desmond Morton (Chairman of the Governors). Behind the Queen is Lord Cottesloe (Chairman of the School Council)

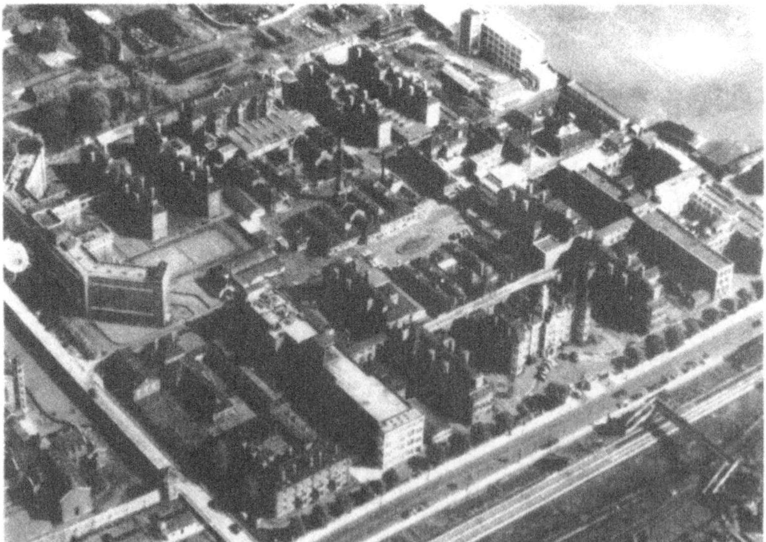

Figure 28 *c.* 1957 Aerial view. Note top right the M.R.C. Cyclotron block of four floors: top left the recruiting huts and trees beyond the hospital site, and below these the new flat-roofed cafeteria where the original dining hall was. Below, the railway lines of the loop line on which 20 years later the Du Cane housing project was to be built

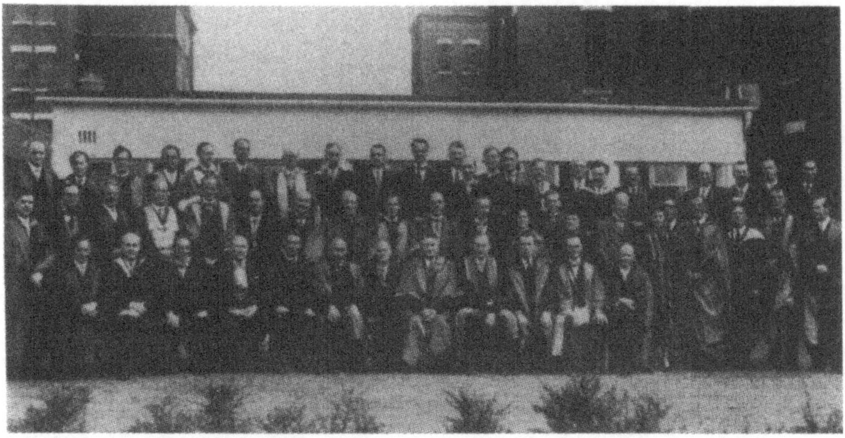

Figure 29 The total consultant staff of the Postgraduate Medical School of London and Hammersmith Hospital in 1957

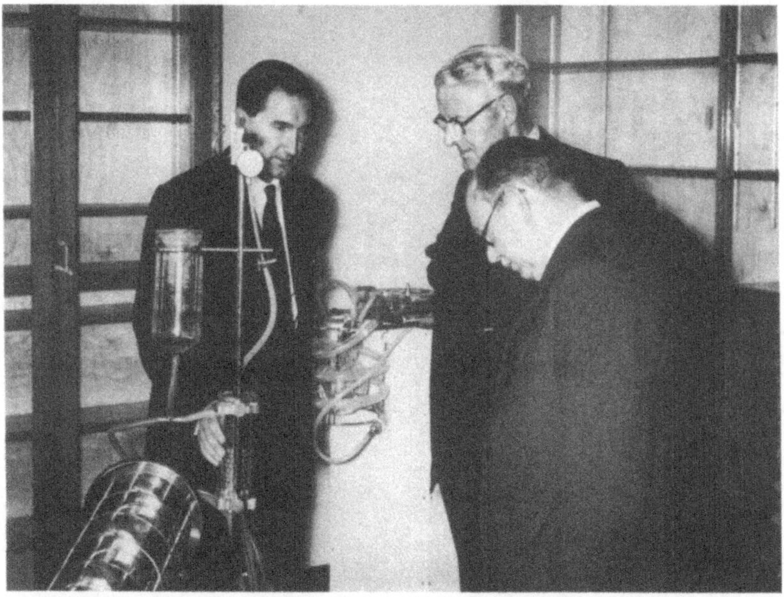

Figure 30 22 June 1959. The opening by Sir James Patterson Ross, President of the Royal College of Surgeons, of the new Surgical Research Laboratories above the Cyclotron Building. Left to right: Melrose (demonstrating his heart–lung machine), Mr W. W. Watt (Treasurer of the School) and Kilner (who had been on the staff of the Hospital in 1918!)

8

The Four Necessities

Four items were considered essential by the Foundation Professors for the development of a successful institute of postgraduate medical education: a library, a workshop, medical photography, and residential accommodation for students. The reasons for each were fairly obvious. Fifty years later all have been acquired: none turned out exactly as planned, but all required generous donors, much imagination and a great deal of perseverance. What many considered the 'fifth necessity' – good public transport – has hardly improved in the half-century.

A LIBRARY

From the earliest days of debate about postgraduate medical education it had always been agreed that any such centre should be close to the great libraries of London: those of the University and the Royal Society of Medicine. The need for a medical library was never questioned; the advantages of a library of the size of the Royal Society of Medicine were acknowledged, the disadvantages never considered. The traditional view was that a university student spent a great deal of his time – perhaps whole days at a time – at this seat of learning, reading books and making notes. No one, when the School was founded 50 years ago, could have conceived the manner in which people at the Hammersmith would use their own library.

The School library evolved to provide specific needs. It remains essentially a library of journals rather than books; the current issues of journals are arranged on racks with bound volumes of the previous 6 years nearby (the earlier editions being in the basement), there is an easy-view catalogue of journals available in alphabetical order with their shelf numbers indicated, and twelve reading tables seating eight persons each. The reader is likely to make frequent, short visits to the library for different purposes: to check a reference, to scan a journal, to prepare for a lecture or patient demonstration. Many diseases span several disparate journals, hence the need to be able to collect these easily for quick reading. Indeed, speed and familiarity with the geography of the library is essential for each specialty. Keeping up-to-date was an attitude acquired early on, because anyone who attempted to teach the teachers must include a daily visit to a library as part of routine mental toilet. It was a place for refreshment, not contemplation.

The Royal Society of Medicine (R.S.M.), probably the largest postgraduate medical research collection in Europe, in February 1984 displayed 2200 current journals, possessed over 450,000 volumes, was laid out on three floors and the average number of daily readers at table was twenty. In the same month and year the Wellcome Library of the Royal Postgraduate Medical School had a daily average of over 250 readers at table (the turnstile, inserted for security in 1978, registered 600 users); it displayed 850 current journals, 7000 bound volumes (80% are journals) and is laid out on one floor, but does offer eight carousels for isolated study on the floor below where older journals are stacked. The R.S.M. Library had become unmanageable for the regular casual reader: the stock too large and too widespread for speedy easy access, a risk that the School recognized.

The School library was started in 1935. Mr G. A. Lloyd was appointed librarian, a library sub-committee of seven members constituted (there were only five people on the Finance and General Purposes Committee, and 13 on the Board of Studies), a site allocated close by the upper lecture room on the first floor of L block (later to become the classroom for the D.C.P. Course), and shelving erected. The proprietors of the *Lancet* presented a complete set of their weekly journal, from its origin in 1823 to date, bound in red half-morocco where it occupied a place of honour at the end of the library, a striking feature of the room. The British Medical Association also presented a complete set of the *British Medical Journal*, and complete sets of various other journals were presented by the Foundation Professors.

Large numbers of periodicals in specialist subjects were taken by subscription: the bill was £414/15/1 in 1936, rising to over £500 in 1938 – roughly 1% of the Treasury Grant to the School (this became the University Grant after a 3-year trial period). In 1936 there were 117 different journals taken regularly, of which six were gifts: in 1939 the figure had risen to 135. In 1937, 106 new books were bought and 93 were presented by staff members, a practice that was encouraged. In the same year 178 volumes of periodicals of previous years were bound and placed on the library shelves; this was good library practice, but did reduce the budget available for new works (reprints and pamphlets – 5500 acquired by 1939 – were stored in boxes).

In 1940 Lloyd was called up for War Service, and the most valuable books – the early bound volumes – were moved by one of the Governors, Mr Goodenough, to his country home to avoid loss from bombing (it never happened, but in May 1941 the Hunterian Museum of the Royal College of Surgeons was badly hit and Grey Turner was moved to comment on the teaching value of his own 'specimens' in glass jars brought from Newcastle). Dorothy Atkins, an experienced librarian, was appointed as a locum for the duration: she resigned before Lloyd returned in 1946, but Lloyd left the following year for 'an important post'. The librarian was paid an annual salary of £253/15/10 in 1936 rising by £10 a year (in 1941 Miss Atkins was paid £292/19/3, the same rate). When Miss Atkins resigned in 1946 she became Medical Librarian to the British Council but was taken back by the School in 1947, where she stayed until retirement in September 1973.

From the beginning it was realized that there would be a limit to the amount spent on the library service. Hence the money should be spent essentially on journals because up-to-date medical advances would be reported there, but the decision was made to subscribe to the National Central Library for the borrowing of books and journals not available locally and to Lewis's Lending Library for textbooks. But for the next 20 years the most pressing need was for a permanent home and enough storage space. One of the army huts erected within the School courtyard was designated for the new library and Miss Wollacott was appointed assistant librarian: she 'resigned on marriage'[57] at the end of 1948 and Miss Jelley from the Chester Beatty Research Institute at the Royal Cancer Hospital (later the Royal Marsden Hospital) took her place. By then, a Medical Section of the Library Association had been formed (in October 1947, another one of Sir William Osler's ideas) and a Scientific Information Conference had been held at the Royal Society in July. As a result, Miss Atkins started a 'Weekly Bulletin' for 50 internal staff. Nothing elaborate but extremely practical: the title, author and page numbers of all the articles published in the periodicals received were typed and duplicated on foolscap sheets, stapled at the top left-hand corner. The journals were listed alphabetically, their contents numerically, so that a reader could either scan all journals and the titles of their articles or be more selective. It was an immediate success and was to be a well-known feature of the library and of the School for nearly 30 years.

The cataloguing and classification of reprints, the checking of references for theses and staff publications, interlibrary loans and internal loans (of 550 a month in 1950) kept the two librarians busy; but it was not until early 1952 that the nearby hut formerly used as the School refectory (discontinued when the Hospital canteen opened) was turned into a reading room. The expansion was short-lived because part of the library hut became the Photographic Department. However, by rearrangement it was possible to seat 64 readers compared with 18 the year before.

In the year of the Jubilee of the Hospital, the library hut exhibited the 23 books written by members of staff and the 25 journals of which staff were either editors or closely concerned with the editing of symposia. In that year the weekly Library Bulletin had 61 external subscribers (usually expatriates of the School) world-wide. The office from which the Bulletin emanated was 12 feet square, lined from floor to ceiling on two sides by journals and books, seated the Librarian and her two assistants, accommodated two typewriters, two telephones and a Tannoy: yet by 1960 there were 232 subscribers, from Helsinki to Honolulu, from Auckland to Yale, more than twice that of the circulation within the School. There was even an arrangement whereby stencils were flown out weekly to the University of Sydney for local reproduction and distribution in Australia.[58]

When the excavations began for the School's Central Laboratory block bound volumes of journals were transferred temporarily to the University library. A photocopier was installed for School staff to use and to copy articles for other libraries to retain. It is often forgotten that there was a brisk trade between borrowers and lenders over many years: in 1948, 215 items were borrowed and 184 lent; 10 years later 851 borrowed, 827 lent. These figures should be compared with internal loans of over 11,500 in 1958 when the Wellcome Trust donated £60,000 to build an entirely new library – eventually to be visited by the Queen in 1966 and admired by all.

The new library in the Commonwealth Building attempted to keep pace with events. All staff in 1984 are graduates, and tend to specialize – periodicals, reader services, inter-library loans (running at over 8000 annually: the National Lending Library at Boston is still the most useful source), and technical services. There is a staff of seven, a photocopier in constant use, facilities for computer searches, the journals are still easy to find and consult, and there are tape–slide programmes as part of an audio-visual aids system. Nearly half the textbooks are donated, and about a third of the periodicals. The library does a job for the staff of School and Hospital and its students which is rarely matched anywhere else. The idea that a library is a place for meditation and solitude was never popular: few of the Foundation Professors could have realized that it would develop into a supermarket rather than a monastery.

A WORKSHOP

At pre-war local authority hospitals the hospital engineer was responsible for the boiler house and the supply of power. He was a professional not a tradesman, and was employed by the local authority not the hospital. It had been thus since the Poor Law days. At Hammersmith Hospital the boiler house was at the centre of the site, the more easily to serve the Infirmary and the Workhouse. Three coal-burning Lancashire boilers, sited below ground, were serviced by stokers (usually ex-navy) who would shift around 1 ton of coal each in an 8-hour shift. Above the boiler house was the laundry; beside it the coal yard. The weighbridge, still present today, was at the west end of the internal road that separated the North Block or Workhouse from the South Block or Infirmary. After the war, when it was clear that the Hospital would need more power, a second-hand boiler was installed nearby, known as Abbott's Folly (in honour of the serving hospital engineer) which blew up in 1957. In preparation for the building of a new hospital a new 'house' for oil-burning boilers (because that was the modern cheap fuel at the time) was built and opened in the north-east corner of the site in 1962. Steam pipes were carried on 20-feet-high steel pillars around the hospital grounds until 1974 when they were laid underground.

The hospital engineer, as befitting his status and needs, also had a workshop often surprisingly well-furnished, including a metal lathe, for repairs to his equipment or the fabrication of new instruments. During the war these workshops were turned over to the production of armaments, for such things as spring covers for tanks, the raw steel cylinders being delivered and the finished articles collected weekly. Most of the work was done after hours by all grades of staff as part of the 'war effort'.

When the School was being built a workshop was included in the request for accommodation: a room on the first floor in L block next to the X-ray department was provided but no engineer appointed, although it was used by School technicians for minor jobs. When the School workshop, which had been in abeyance during the war because its lathe was lent to the Government for war-work, was re-instituted in 1947, a whole-time technician (Con Lordan) was appointed and Dr C. Wood was Medical Engineer-in-charge. A number of new machine tools were purchased from surplus Government stores and the whole workshop re-equipped pending the time when a new workshop could be built for the joint use of the London County Council (that is the hospital engineer's separate workshop) and the School. The Annual Report for 1947 commented: 'This project is a new departure and is an attempt to economise on the existing arrangement under which there are three separate workshops on site (the third was in radiotherapy). By co-operating with the L.C.C. it is hoped to provide a much better-equipped workshop for the combined use of the Physics Department of the L.C.C. The temporary restarting of the School workshop has already proved the great value of facilities to construct research apparatus for the use of professional staff.'

What the School had in mind was for a workshop to make 'standard' equipment and save money. What no one envisaged at the time was the potential for making new and pilot equipment that no one else in the world could make, or dared to take the risk of making commercially and suffering financial losses. Many pieces of original design, usually the brainchild of an experimentalist on the staff, were fabricated under difficult conditions. Lordan was paid a wage of £398/2/6 in 1948, just half the salary of the librarian.

In the following year the School took a pioneer step in forming a Department of Biophysics – arguing that biophysics was about 30 years behind biochemistry yet full of potential – and appointed David Hill as Senior Lecturer to take up his duties in 1949. He was offered a small office in the Lower Medical Corridor (the wooden hut which had been hastily erected soon after the School opened in 1935; the building survives in 1984). This was the first move to establish a division of medical engineering and architects were asked to design a new building to accommodate the workshop and biophysics. In 1951 the new building, leading off the North corridor between H and I blocks, came into use and in 1956 an electronics section was added, run by John Gilbert (followed by John Fox in 1961) with two senior electronic engineers. Lordan likewise recruited two extra mechanics as 'instrument makers', a recognized trade for the kind of person required. The first joint project was the construction of a mass spectrometer for rapid gas analysis (the prototype devised by Fowler) which was used to study lung function in normal and diseased patients.

In 1959 the Cambridge Instrument Company funded the post of an additional lecturer in Electronics Engineering (Pallett from Edinburgh was appointed): Dr G. R. Ball, a qualified engineer and physician, had been made a full-time lecturer the previous year. Together they supervised the designs of many new instruments as well as providing technical advice to all staff. In the next 10 years a variety of instruments were invented and made: not all were successful, but all were exciting.

When Sir Isaac Wolfson donated money for a building to provide 'amenities' (dining rooms and lecture theatres) and laid the foundation stone in 1959 the School was quick to include a basement floor of nearly 750 square metres for a new workshop and electronic laboratory, the whole to constitute a department of mechanical and electrical engineering. The basement workshop of the Wolfson Institute became a showpiece for visitors to the School: there was nothing quite like it anywhere else in the world.

In 1966 there were as many as twenty instrument makers engaged on a range of inventions which varied from the smallest blood flow measuring catheter (to be inserted into the umbilical artery of premature babies, for the paediatric unit) to a low-level swivel stool and automatic film changer (for taking serial X-rays of blood vessels for the Department of Radiology), from an experimental mitral valve for replacement cardiac surgery to an integral-hinge artificial finger joint for replacement reconstructive hand surgery – both being produced in extrusion moulds from polypropylene – a metabolic cage for rats, a one-handed needle holder, an extra thin silicone rubber film for differential filtration, the Melrose oxygenator, heat-exchangers, an anaesthetic mask for mice. The list was endless. The mechanical instruments were produced in one workshop and the electrical components next door. Such items as an eight-channel recorder could not be bought on the open market and although the district around the Hammersmith was choc-a-bloc with small engineering companies none was either prepared or capable of producing what various staff members wanted.

The system worked like this. The researcher – for the workshop was essentially to do with research and inventions – would draw what he wanted or thought he wanted on the back of an envelope and then discuss his requirements with the technician-in-charge. The latter would listen with pencil in hand to make his own drawing (on the back of another envelope if necessary) to make sure that minds and ideas were in tune. At a meeting a week or so later the customer would be presented with a proper engineer's drawing with measurements and perspective. If he approved that drawing – many people failed to recognize their own invention at that stage – then the instrument would be made by Stan, or Jim, or David, or by any one of the company who was available or who had the necessary special skills. The article was often made in brass, a soft metal which was cheap, easy to work and easy to modify: the customer took it away and if it 'worked', that is it did what the inventor expected it to do after a reasonable trial, the article was returned to the workshop for chrome-plating. The final product looked good, did a job, and was unique.

The presence of a well-equipped workshop (there were six lathes, four drilling machines, metal guillotines, ovens, drawing boards, and numerous power tools) on site and capable of making almost anything was not only a stimulus to the inventor but facilitated the acquisition of new knowledge. For instance, as already mentioned, the first mass spectrometer designed by Hill and Fowler was made in the School Workshop. The use of this, together with short-life oxygen isotopes piped from the M.R.C. cyclotron to the laboratory, allowed measurement of the concentration of gases in the alveoli of the lungs. The discovery that there was differential damage to the apex of the lung in mitral stenosis was not only a stimulus to those developing cardiac surgery to get on with it and save lives (Melrose was working on an oxygenator for an artificial lung at Downe – Charles Darwin's old home in Kent – under difficult conditions at the time and had already decided to stop the heart with potassium to allow the surgeon to make the necessary reconstruction with a 'still heart'), but also the solution to a puzzle that astute physicians had known for nearly a century: patients with mitral stenosis did not suffer from apical pulmonary tuberculosis, yet both were common in their time. The School's findings were condemned by the pundits of the day as 'non-scientific' because the work could not be repeated by others who did not have the necessary equipment to do so! A nice point of pusillanimity.[59]

It is impossible to over-estimate the value of the service to the staff of School and Hospital. The set-up was ideal for inventors. There was even a consultant (Dr Ball, a G.P., but qualified engineer and adviser to Vickers) available to give advice on the more theoretical and difficult problems. There were no forms to fill in, at least not at first, and both engineer and clinician understood what the tool was to do, had the same interest in making sure that it was right for the job. As a result many practical advances were made. It was only in the seventies, when economies demanded repayment for all services rendered, that grant monies had to be found to cover the cost of each instrument maker. By 1984 the workshop complement had been reduced to six. Con Lordan retired in 1979 (and died a year later) but the tradition of service, dedication, perfection and mutual satisfaction lived on. It was never quite clear why the School in 1935 was so keen on having its own workshop, which became a unique feature of the Hammersmith and was never copied by any other school in London, but there is little doubt that the workshop was the envy of researchers working at other institutions world-wide.

Curiously, the Hospital set up its own instrument workshop in 1960 (under Freddy Dewar) to repair equipment. By 1984 this unit had expanded to a staff of three who are fully occupied and are a source of savings for the N.H.S. as well as an example to other hospitals of the value of such an enterprise.

PHOTOGRAPHY

The School pioneered medical photography and cultivated its growth. The Foundation Professors wanted their own photographic unit for two reasons: the clinicians wanted slides and prints as records of unusual patients and the pathologists of their histology: both were needed for teaching and publications. The first photographer, Mr V. V. Wilmott, was appointed in 1938 and his dark-room was at the south-west side of the School building on the ground floor conveniently close to the post-mortem room. The annual report recorded: 'The School photographer is in constant demand in preparing slides and diagrams, etc., for lectures and the work of his department has much increased'. Grey Turner had brought John Robson, his technician, from Newcastle when he came in 1935 and Robson had illustrated Turner's own textbook with half-tone drawings: Robson was an accomplished artist and did much drawing in the School as well as organizing the routine technical services in the Department of Surgery.

The photographer (who was also slide-projectionist at staff rounds and lectures) was paid a wage of £290/9/3 in 1941, just £60 more than the salary of the librarian, and the next year took an assistant. By 1947 the wages for photography (£1490) exceeded the total for the librarian's salary, assistant's wages, and cost of journals by £170. Photography had grown rapidly.

In the 1946 report the Dean wrote: 'The School has been a pioneer in the application of photography to medicine and has demonstrated the great value of this adjunct to teaching and research. The Department is repeatedly visited by representatives of other schools desirous of learning how to set up a department of their own. As an ancillary to the Photographic Department, the appointment of a part-time medical artist proved so successful that this year a full-time artist, Miss Helen Wilson, was appointed'. The Department was very cramped in the 'studio' on the ground floor and 'had extended into rooms leased from the London County Council because of the considerable increase in staff'. When war came such luxuries as medical photography were reduced, but in 1951 Wilmott was made a Fellow of the Institute of British Photographers for his services to medical photography.

During the post-war austerity, part of the library reading room – the old School refectory hut – was turned over to photography and soon the Department was producing films. In 1955 the first full-length epic, 'Bilateral Adrenalectomy by the Anterior Abdominal Approach', was touring the U.S.A. and Canada; the U.S.A. had also purchased two copies of 'Portal Systemic Encephalopathy'. The next year the second sound film was produced – 'Arterial Grafting' – in spite of the work involved in producing displays for the tercentenary celebrations of William Harvey (the discoverer of the circulation) both at Hammersmith and at the Royal College of Physicians in Pall Mall. Eleven members of staff had left in the previous decade to become principals elsewhere, so that frequent changes of personnel added to the difficulties of cramped quarters – filming had to be done at week-ends – and an increasing volume of work. Two films were made the following year – 'The Use of the Artificial Kidney' and 'The Effective Myometrial Blood Flow' – and the British Council bought 10 copies of an earlier film ('Vaginal Hysterectomy') for distribution abroad.

By 1957 the School was considered to be the major producer of medical films in the U.K. (other than sponsored films) and they were the speciality of Brecknell, head of the Department. There was also a change from 3¼ inch square slides to 35 mm as the standard format, in the expectation that there would be less work involved. No one predicted the explosion in quantity that such a change was to set off; 10 years later in 1967 the Department produced over 15,000 prints and the same number of slides, a figure that was to double again in the following decade.

By 1959 rationing of requests for medical illustration became inevitable, and ineffective. Staff increased but so did demand. In that year the new Experimental Surgical Laboratories were opened by Sir Henry Dale (on 22 June) for which an exhibition of photographs and art work, demonstrating the research in the School, was mounted on 23 panels. The big change came with the introduction of colour film for slides at the time of the opening of the new and additional lecture theatres in the Wolfson Building. A third projectionist was appointed and bookings for the use of a lecture theatre had to be made formally: within 10 years bookings would be made nearly a year ahead, such was the demand. Films were still being made and in 1962 'The Emergency Treatment of Cardiac Arrest' (38 copies were sold worldwide in the next 5 years) and 'Neonatal Care' were first screened in Australia. When the Department moved to premises in the newly built and enlarged Medical School in 1966 it was assumed that filming would be a major activity: a large studio, a special projection room for single-person viewing, and much modern equipment were provided. Luxury indeed, and with it a sudden cessation of demand. No further films were made until 1972: one on nitrous oxide anaesthesia and another on muscle biopsy. The filming days were virtually over. In the reorganization of the School in 1982, when the three separate units of photomicrography, clinical photography, and graphics were united onto smaller premises on the same floor, the film studio was put to other use.

The number of courses and seminars had increased markedly in the seventies so that three full-time projectionists were employed, but it was clear that there had to be a change to automatic machines for slides (with the lecturer controlling the rate of projection of his own slides: hardly any lectures were given without slides) and manual facilities – the School had won an enviable reputation in lecture theatre techniques – being reserved for the great occasions. The demand for lecture theatres continued and most were upgraded by the addition of new equipment. The increasing demand for slides, partly due to the increasing speed of presentation of computerized results in research and mainly of graphics, had been growing since 1974: prior to that the medical artist turned out about 2000 pieces of work annually, but in that year there was a 68% increase to 3220 pieces, a very significant change in current practice.

From the earliest days medical illustration had been fostered as a discipline necessary to support high-quality lectures and publications at home and abroad, to illustrate the new and unusual, to convey concepts and understanding. Initially photography was the essential tool and line work was done by a chartist, a rather boring job which failed to retain a competent worker for any length of time. Most illustrations were half-tone and often for textbooks. At one time chartists were moving through the Department at the same 6-monthly turnover rate as medical housemen and even the introduction of better equipment did not help. The problem in the early seventies was obvious: too many people wanted too many line illustrations, particularly graphs and charts, for too many uses although publication was the prime need. Doig Simmonds introduced a do-it-yourself drawing board, instructions, free materials, freely available advice from a professional artist, and out-of-hours working: he then obtained cheap, quick prints and passable slides on an automatic machine to reduce the demand for professional photography which was likely to follow any increased productivity. The scheme was introduced in 1975 and at first attracted only those pushy juniors who previously had had difficulty in obtaining the services, or even the advice, of a medical artist.

The production figures read like those of a go-ahead commercial company. In 1975 the do-it-yourself clinicians and secretaries completed on average 250 items of work monthly, about 3000 annually: in 1977 it was 500 and in 1979 (and for the next 3 years remained at) 700 monthly, a total of over 8000 annually, or equal to the output of three full-time chartists which the School could neither afford nor retain. There were 80 users in 1975 and 180 in 1981, but the value of the scheme was only appreciated when one looked at the variation in monthly totals – a feature that no chartist can accommodate – which were well-recognized at Hammersmith as the 'panic months' that preceded the mounting of specialist courses and where rank and status were essential for the delivery of precious slides on time. In 1981 the monthly output varied from 330 in January to 890 in March and April out of a total of 8400 items. Clearly the D.I.Y. system of flexible working was successful in number, and has been taken up by the World Health Organization which currently pays for courses in developing countries. What of quality? No one could tell the difference between the level of work of an experienced amateur and the professional artist: what was lost on skill was made up on devotion. Moreover, new techniques for automatic photography, to produce slides and prints of acceptable quality 'while-you-wait' were being developed universally in the eighties so that the Hammersmith now had a Department of Medical Illustration in the true sense and not just a group of expert photographers. It seems likely that computer graphics, showing three-dimensional drawings from any perspective, and available to architects in 1984, will become equally popular in medicine. The beauty of the D.I.Y. system was that output matched demand because demand had become self-regulating, in the same way that photomicrography had become a personal skill with the advent of light and exposure controls fitted to the cameras made for the pathologists' microscopes in 1967: almost overnight the production of slides of microscopy became simple and satisfactory.

HOUSING FOR STUDENTS

The report of the Athlone Committee in 1921 had recommended that there should be a postgraduate medical school in the centre of London, with a central office to co-ordinate teaching, and 'a library, hostel, and everything necessary to afford full facilities for social intercourse'. And further, 'A hostel for the convenience of doctors attending the courses from a distance would be desirable. We attach considerable importance to the social side of the scheme and think that one of its chief merits will be in the opportunity for intercourse and discussion between the graduates themselves.' The Postgraduate Medical Education Committee, set up in 1925 and reporting in 1930, recorded that 'the provision of a residential hostel for postgraduate students is an indispensable element in the scheme. A residential hostel does not exist at the Hammersmith Hospital, and the cost of building and equipping such a hostel must accordingly be accepted as an inevitable part of the capital cost of the conversion of the Hospital.' The Committee emphasized that by providing hostel accommodation this would also 'overcome, or at least mitigate, an objection which may be felt to the Hammersmith Hospital, namely, the distance at which the Hospital stands from the medical centre of London'. Residential facilities should 'be provided as part of the fabric of the British Postgraduate Hospital and Medical School'.

The recommendation had been incorporated in the Royal Charter of 1931, for the Governing Body 'to provide, or arrange for the provision of, residential facilities in London for students of the School'. But to no avail. When the recession of the thirties came, and the risk of abandonment of the whole project seemed inevitable and funds were reduced by half, the new Nurses Home was built; student residencies were not. Students were accommodated in University lodgings in Bloomsbury but found the distance to travel inconvenient. Several schemes were debated but in the recession after the war the priority was to develop the School and Hospital.

It was not until Taylor was appointed Dean, and Vellacott School Secretary, in 1965, that a concerted attempt was made to solve the problem of overseas student accommodation. London was becoming more expensive and more crowded, and there was some evidence that the lack of suitable rooms nearby was affecting overseas student numbers: there had been a 10% drop in the past 5 years. Besides, with a much larger new medical school and new facilities the demand was likely to be greater.

In 1965 the School joined AFSIL Ltd (Accommodation for Students in London) and with the London School of Economics, the London School of Hygiene and Tropical Medicine, the School of Oriental and African Studies, and University College planned to provide postgraduate accommodation. AFSIL had about 60 dwellings of which the School had an option on 12, but they were inconveniently sited: the School also joined SRC Ltd (Student Residential Centres), who had shown interest in providing accommodation expressly for Hammersmith postgraduates. There was no progress for 3 years until the British Railways Board and the London Transport Executive declared a small strip of land on the south side of Du Cane road to be 'surplus to their requirements': the land had been a rubbish tip in the last century and then a loop for a main-line railway, but the proximity to the Hammersmith Hospital and School attracted interest.

The School invited AFSIL and SRC to co-operate to purchase the land and develop it; after 3 years of negotiations the scheme was abandoned. However, on 15 July 1970 Lord Aberdare, Minister of State for the Department of Health and Social Services (D.H.S.S.) spoke to the House of Lords about Housing Associations and postgraduate students. He said, 'I can say today that we accept straight away one suggestion, that has been put forward, that housing associations for married postgraduate students should be eligible for the same subsidies as other housing associations entering into arrangements with their local authority.' This statement prompted Lord Coleraine, Chairman of the School Council, to set up a small group (Sir Leon Bagrit, David Rhodes, Pat Matthews and George Vellacott) to try to buy the land on-

Du Cane Road; the group co-opted Harold Campbell, an expert and pioneer in housing associations.

In March 1972 the Du Cane Housing Association was formed with 10 foundation members and registered as a charity with the Registrar of Friendly Societies. In October the First National Finance Corporation (Pat Matthews) granted a bridging loan of £157,000 because planning permission to develop the land had not yet been obtained. A further feasibility study and soil exploration was undertaken by the architects 'at their own risk' so that they could be sure the Parker Morris standards (of the accommodation to be provided) and the Department of Environment yardsticks (of the appearance and substance of the building) would apply if the Housing Association obtained a loan from the Greater London Council (G.L.C.) to build. Both of these 'standards' were being enforced in all council house buildings.

At the time the Housing Finance Act of 1973 had not been approved by Parliament. Even so, calculations in 1972 showed that the completed project would run at an annual loss of £15,000 for about 10 years. In addition, money would have to be raised to furnish the rooms and this could not come from a G.L.C. loan. The loan was granted in August, but not taken up because planning permission was not received from Hammersmith Borough Council until May 1973. Permission to build was then turned down by the Department of the Environment on the grounds of too high density and a lack of amenities: both were conditions that students would welcome as aids to study. After 6 months of further negotiations permission was granted in January 1974. In September the G.L.C. loan was taken up and the First National Finance Corporation repaid, and in December the architects, quantity surveyors and solicitors received their first payments for 4 years of painstaking negotiations, detailed work and many frustrations.

The contract was awarded in October to build 112 residencies for between £1.9 million and £2.5 million. Work started in January 1975 and the five blocks of flats were handed over in April 1977. In order to provide professional expertise and management for the Du Cane Housing Association the Co-ownership Development Society (of Balham) was appointed, but did not come up to expectations; the contract was terminated in May 1977. Instead, the School took over management and Vellacott became secretary to the Du Cane Housing Association. When the Housing Act of 1974 became law, the Association registered with the Housing Corporation and was relieved of the necessity to find money for the expected annual deficit, subject to audit and good management. The Act required the Association to charge not more than 'fair rents' (as determined by the Hammersmith Borough Rent Service Officer). The Act also gave the local authority the right to 50% of the available housing to be allocated to persons nominated by them. Generously, the G.L.C. waived their rights under the Act, thus allowing the School 100% right of accommodation.

Appropriately, the opening ceremony on 13 October 1977 was performed by Lord Pitt of Hampstead in Greater London and Grenada. Created a life peer in 1975, Lord Pitt qualified as a doctor from Edinburgh University, had served in public health in the West Indies, had been in general practice since 1947 and was currently Chairman of the Community Relations Commission.

The whole enterprise had taken exactly 12 years: it had occupied the entire duration of Taylor as Dean, Vellacott as School Secretary: it had demonstrated the value of courage, friends and tenacity: it allowed students to bring their families from abroad and live cheaply in London: it also provided the School with the ability to invite and accommodate a visiting Professor within the environment of the campus: it was an immediate success from the start and for the first time brought to the Hammersmith a resident student population. In 1981 a total of 842 postgraduates attended the School (a University full-time equivalent student number of 505) of whom 223 were eligible to be nominated for accommodation with the Du Cane Housing Association. In February 1982 there was a Housing Corporation Monitoring visit: the monitors were impressed with what they saw. The final settlement of all accounts was £3.4 million: of this £3 million was Housing Association Grant leaving the Du Cane Housing Association with a mortgage to the G.L.C. of about £½ million repayable over 60 years. The appeal for funds launched in the early days netted £151,000, which paid for furnishings.

In the first 5 years 530 students were accommodated 'across the road' in the 48 one-bedroomed flats and 64 three-bedroomed maisonettes. Most were accompanied by their families from abroad and there were usually around 100 children in residence at any given time. The vast majority of these post-graduate student tenants were outspoken in their appreciation both of the accommodation offered and the service provided.

9

Growth: the Bare Essentials (1945–1966)

Every organization, no matter how small and simple or large and complex, uses resources to achieve its aims. These resources can be categorized broadly under four main headings: space, people, materials and machines. This concept is universal and applies to any kind of enterprise, whether it be commercial or professional; it certainly applied to the post-war Hammersmith and all four were pursued when opportunities arose.

The aims of the pre-war School (recorded in Chapter 4) had been changed by the 1947 Charter: from now on the Federation would look after the postgraduate education of doctors intended for general practice – more than half the output from the undergraduate medical schools – and would cover certain specialist subjects. Hammersmith was, therefore, freed to develop something unique. The post-war Professors wanted research to become a part of normal life at the Hammersmith. They wished to inoculate the doctors on the staff with the contagion of scientific curiosity, to see it spread, to encourage all doctors to bring the problems of their patients to the laboratory and to use the insights of scientific method at the bedside. They set about finding space, gathering funds, and most importantly, assembling a group of promising young men who were often sent away to other medical centres for special training in preparation of the task ahead. By general consensus it was decided that new building was the prime necessity.

The gross space of about 14 acres was unlikely to be enlarged although there was the old army recruiting ground at the back which had served two world wars and now was derelict. In the sixties an attempt was made to acquire the site, but since it had originally been part of the common land further north, an

Act of Parliament would have been required (and the costs debited to the School) to acquire it from 'The People'; the idea was abandoned. Even before war started the School was overcrowded. Clearly new building was required, but the country's need was for houses not labs and there were shortages of materials. Even so, plans were laid in the early fifties (it should be remembered that bread rationing was introduced for the first time in 1947, and wartime sweet rationing did not cease until 1954).

HUTTED EXPANSION

The 1945 Government's scheme for further education of demobilized doctors, in the form of supernumerary registrarships, began in August and peaked in October. It had been expected that the teachers would be the first to be released, and that the potential students would follow: in fact, it was found that, because the services had to retain a good many specialists for the time being (because of the fear of a new conflict), it was the officers in need of further education who were demobilized first. This threw a strain on the teaching staff of the School, to which they responded with enthusiasm. The real trouble was that there was no room for the influx. However, Aneurin Bevan, the then Minister of Health, visited the School in January 1946 and arranged for licences to be granted for the erection of eight Army huts which the L.C.C. allowed to be put on their land. The University advanced the necessary funds, building started in the summer but was not completed until the next year. The appalling weather during the winter, and for the Spring of 1947 when thick snow lay in many parts of London until the end of March, delayed construction.

The eight huts were erected at the back of the School: library, records room (a Records officer was appointed by the School because the Hospital records of patients were not considered sufficient and School records were thought to be valuable 'seed-corn' for future research: Mr B. B. Bonner was appointed to take charge), animal house, common rooms, Department of Medicine offices (the Department of Surgery was at the other end of the South Corridor of the Hospital, in the old operating theatre and X-ray room: where the Intensive Care block now stands), and a stores hut. The hut for offices for Surgery and that for Obstetrics and Gynaecology were not able to be occupied because no telephones were installed. Even in the library there was no heating until January 1948. It was a time of acute shortages at home as well as financial crises abroad: the Marshall Plan for Aid to Europe had just been launched in an attempt to dispel the doom and gloom.

In 1945 there were 96 students and Registrars in the Department of Medicine alone: twenty of these were accommodated at Redhill County Hospital (Middlesex County Council) and St James' Hospital (L.C.C.), who came to the Hammersmith for the Wednesday Clinico-pathological conference, but it was not a satisfactory arrangement and clearly something had to be done.

In 1948 a new animal house was built on the roof of the Pathology Department which had began to expand and occupy more and more of the original School building (the complete 'occupation' occurred in 1966). By converting the old library into a general teaching laboratory and by using former store-rooms, the class for the Academic Diploma in Clinical Pathology numbered 20 for the first time. This course of instruction, one of the more important for home and overseas doctors, had an interesting history. The Diploma was first awarded in 1930, but up to 1937 only eight candidates had presented themselves for examination (and only five diplomas awarded). The 1-year course was to become the most popular at Hammersmith, with demand exceeding accommodation for the next 20 years. But the continual rearranging of accommodation which was to be a distinctive feature of the School for evermore – if only because people and ideas were continually changing – could not be tolerated for long in the cramped quarters provided.

SCHOOL BUILDING FUND

The School building fund was launched in 1956 under the Chairmanship of Mr W. W. Watt, Chairman of a large industrial enterprise (British Oxygen) and an entrepreneur by nature, who was co-opted to the Committee of Management. Mr T. B. H. Ellis produced sketch plans of a completed School. The original Appeal Committee (Professor Aird, Lord Cottesloe, Professor Dible, Dr Fletcher and the Dean) spent the summer planning and preparing an appeal brochure and then enlarged the committee by 11 more members; the Earl of Athlone became the Patron and a body of 12 distinguished persons the sponsors. The Appeal was launched by a special article in *The Times* on 31 October 1956, a Press Conference next day, and articles in the *Lancet* and *British Medical Journal* on 2 November. It was unfortunate that the 'Suez Crisis' started the same week, when a combined Anglo-French force landed in Egypt and grabbed all the headlines. By July 1957 £315,000 had been subscribed.

The appeal had been for a new central laboratory block but in December Mr Isaac Wolfson[60] donated £125,000 for a complete lecture theatre and common-room block – the School badly needed both – and Mr Ellis, the architect, drew up separate plans for this building. The foundation stone was laid by Isaac Wolfson on 2 June 1959 and opened by Harold Macmillan, the Prime Minister, on 3 May 1961. The Wolfson Institute, as it was called, provided three lecture theatres (of seating capacity 75, 140 and 450), a spacious open-plan restaurant, galleries, common rooms, and in the basement two workshops, for biophysics and mechanical engineering: 2350 m^2 of valuable teaching area.

The Wolfson Institute was not the first new building on the School site. At the end of 1950 the Medical Research Council (M.R.C.) started a project in the north-east corner of the grounds, to house a cyclotron (to the north) and a linear accelerator (to the south) on the ground floor with three floors of laboratories for radiobiology research. Because the cyclotron would make radio-isotopes on site (which could not be produced in the pile at Harwell) and these were likely to help in the diagnosis and treatment of disease, the Hospital agreed to build a fourth floor using endowment money. This move by the Hospital set a precedent for 'opportunistic building' which was to cause trouble later. By 1951 the 2-million volt electrostatic generator, built by the M.R.C. staff, was in full operation as a source of electron, neutron and X-ray radiation, and the 8-million volt travelling wave linear accelerator (the first supervoltage machine of its kind ever to be put to clinical use) was completed. The building of three additional floors on top of the M.R.C. Cyclotoron Building, financed by the Wellcome Trust and the University, to be used for experimental surgery and the housing of large animals, started in September 1957; the M.R.C. decided to add another floor for their own use, and these floors were opened by Sir James Patterson Ross, President of the Royal College of Surgeons, on 22 June 1959, after seemingly endless delays.

It now became possible to house those 'out-sections' of experimental work which had been accommodated at the Buxton Browne Farm at Downe, the property of the Royal College of Surgeons. A whole team had been established at that research laboratory since 1950; Dempster transplanting the kidney and Melrose devising the extracorporeal circulation, with visits for shorter projects by Bentall, Shackman, Graber, Daniels and Aird. This new Experimental Surgery Unit (E.S.U.) on three floors of 1200 m^2 also offered bench space to the many in the Department of Medicine who lacked such facilities, although two floors of offices and laboratories had been built over the South Kitchen of the Hospital – close by the B wards medical block and so creating a clinical research centre in that area – and opened on 9 April 1957 as the Francis Fraser Laboratories of 470 m^2 space: these necessary laboratories had been paid for from the School's reserves but needed a generous donation from the British Postgraduate Federation funds to complete them. Sir Harold Himsworth,[61] Secretary of the Medical Research Council, formally opened the building and paid tribute to Sir Francis Fraser, the first Professor of Medicine at the School (who was present), and to his leadership in making the two vital decisions which set the School on the road to distinction, 'a centre of medical thought rather than a mere coaching establishment'. Himsworth continued: 'the first [decision] was that this school should make its reputation on its ability to advance knowledge . . . many questioned whether that was your prime function; they were people who thought that your major effort should have been to organise refresher courses or cram courses for higher degrees. That this did not happen is largely due to the convictions and firmness of one man. The second decision was that from the start not only the School but also the Hospital should be organised on classical University lines . . . some few years ago one of the men who had been most critical admitted to me that your new School would never have achieved so much so rapidly had it not adopted this pattern or organisation.' In the same year Professor McMichael was elected to the Fellowship of the Royal Society, a signal honour for a physician, official recognition of modern clinical science as practised at the Hammersmith.

Early in 1960, Watt, the original chairman, retired and the Building Appeal, now standing at £645,000, was temporarily halted: Lord Coleraine, Professor Dible, Professor Lord Stamp and Professor King[62] had travelled the world for funds; and Britain's finances were unsteady. However, by April 1962 the fund had risen to £945,000, which made it possible to place the order for the first five floors. Clearly it was desirable to complete the building, up to the eighth floor as planned originally and in one operation, so the Finance Committee restarted the Appeal. Professor Lord Stamp took charge in February 1963. Generous support was forthcoming: one anonymous donor who advertised in *The Times* that he would give to a suitable cause, donated £50,000! By July, Lord Stamp[63] assured the School that the new building could be completed in one stage.

THE BUILDING OF A NEW SCHOOL

On 31 December 1962 the building contractor took over the site, demolished the existing one-storey Works Building and burnt the wooden huts. It was the worst winter for a decade and there were not enough lorries to cart away the excavated clay when digging started in earnest. The original plan allowed money for shoring-up the sides of the deep hole (which was the site of a daily lunch-time pilgrimage for many) but the builder considered this unnecessary until one Friday afternoon, when work had finished for the week, a main waterpipe fractured and rapidly turned the hole into a lake. Tactfully the Dean reported the delay as due to unusually wet weather. There were other delays in this building of cast concrete. The wooden shutterings for each wall took most of the week to erect around steel rods and ties, and the liquid cement was poured between them on a Thursday or Friday so that the cement would set over the week-end and allow work to start next Monday morning. Unfortunately, that winter, there was not a single frost-free night until 6 March 1963. Moreover the plywood shuttering was not strong enough to retain the weight of cement. As a result, when the shuttering was removed on Monday mornings the new-cast wall was bulging and of poor quality; for the next few days the site was clothed in the sound of pneumatic drills removing the previous week's work.

By April the weather and building techniques had improved. On 24 May 1963, Commonwealth Day (in 1966, moved to 11 June), the foundation stone was laid by Field Marshal the Rt Hon. Earl Alexander of Tunis, President of the School. By July the central tower cranes were installed and the vast concrete foundations of the sub-basement completed. The real building had started. In November 1963 the building was 15 weeks behind expectations, and in spite of an unusually mild winter, the slippage reached 32 weeks in July 1964. The original date of completion was to be May 1965, a larger intake of postgraduates was to be made in September and the opening ceremony was planned for April 1966.

During 1965 it was decided that, by certain economies, it would be possible to add another floor: later the Max Rayne Foundation and the Wellcome Trust both made generous benefactions for yet another floor. The ninth floor was to be for Cardiovascular and Pharmacological Research and the tenth floor for Surgical Research.

For the first time, in 1965, a budgeted deficit on the year's working of the School could not be wiped out by care and economy without damaging whole research projects, and a new effort was made to restore the balance: the main causes had been rises in wages awarded by Whitley Councils, and new advances in clinical medicine which had increased the manpower on site. The revised date for occupation of the new building, December 1965, carried a special meaning for the Dean.

Charles Newman had joined the School as Sub-Dean on 31 March 1938 from King's College Hospital and Medical School where he was Physician and Sub-Dean. Newman[64] and Constance O'Driscoll,[65] who had been respectively Acting Dean and Secretary during the war, were appointed Dean and Secretary in 1946. They had worked together for 20 years and seen the School grow materially and spiritually. Both retired in 1965. Charles Newman had a rather disarming addiction to the old-fashioned wing-collar, he addressed people by their surname and without title rather like the housemaster at a Public School, but when he left he could look around with pride: all the gleaming new buildings were School, all the old were Hospital.

THE OFFICIAL OPENING

Queen Elizabeth II opened the new Commonwealth Building on 6 May 1966 (the building was not completely occupied until July when the Department of Surgery moved into the tenth floor: see Appendix I). Her Majesty was received by the President of the School, Field Marshal Earl Alexander of Tunis, and the Major of the Borough of Hammersmith. They proceeded to the large lecture theatre (now called the Stamp Theatre) in the Wolfson Institute where, in the presence of a most distinguished group of visitors and staff in academic gowns, the official opening address was delivered. Her Majesty unveiled a plaque in the entrance hall, toured laboratories, library, offices, was introduced to heads of departments and to a group of principal donors, before taking tea with students from many parts of the world. Most of the Commonwealth High Commissioners were present to meet the Queen and to talk to doctors from their own countries. Lord Coleraine, Chairman of the School, and Lord Cottesloe, Chairman of the Hospital and of the Governing Body of the Federation, said goodbye to Her Majesty at the conclusion of an historic and enjoyable visit.

A NEW HOSPITAL?

During this time the Board of Governors of the Hospital were not idle. The demand was for the construction of a new hospital, in stages, to replace the old. Unfortunately some fundamental thinking was subvented to financial consideration: the question 'how much can we spend?' replaced 'what do we want?'

Walter Gropius, like Corbusier one of the 'modern' architects and educators, believed that all design should be approached in the same way (whether wheelchair, hospital, or city): by a systematic study of needs and problems, taking account of modern construction, materials and techniques, without reference to previous forms and styles. But Medicine is ever changing and it is difficult to forecast changes that lie ahead. Doctors invariably call for flexibility in planning which is really only practicable if the hospital is constructed entirely on a ground floor level and if the wards and the special investigatory departments are so designed that they can be readily extended. Flexibility in a multi-storey construction is not impossible, but is so expensive as to be unwarrantable unless changes can be clearly seen in advance; on the other hand single-storey construction requires a great deal of land on a level site. Nowadays the growing points of a hospital are the pathology and X-ray departments, the out-patient clinics and the casualty department: changes in wards occur much more slowly. Modern ward design usually included about 20% of single rooms, the remainder being divided into bays of four to six patients. Hence it was reasonable to place wards in a monobloc while installing the growing departments in single- or two-storey buildings. The Nuffield Provincial Hospitals Trust architectural teams had designed large ward floors of 30–40 beds on the 'race-track' principle arranged in bays around the central services: they are less popular than they once were and have many disadvantages.

Curiously, the School when it was largely a hutted complex had great flexibility without realizing it. The current hospital likewise could be altered in shape to suit medical requirements, yet the buildings that both School and Hospital expected were tall, not broad, both aimed for linking multi-storey designs. The Board of Governors of the Hospital recognized that upgrading buildings was just as important as new building, however desirable the latter.

In 1951 Professor Basil Ward,[66] of Messrs Ramsey, Murray and White, was employed to devise an overall plan for the complete rebuilding of the Hospital and School so that all future structural developments could be directed towards a predetermined end. Although the chance seemed remote at the time, the idea of a master plan for the site was good. In the event it was ignored. By 1954 the idea of total reconstruction of the Hospital had been abandoned, to be replaced by a plan of renovation of existing buildings. During that year the Governors provided a Metabolic Unit of eight beds and laboratories at the north end of the medical wards: like the B block clinic rooms and the Cyclotron Building, these were the work of Professor Basil Ward.

THE HOSPITAL JUBILEE

The principal event of 1955 was the celebration of the fiftieth anniversary of the opening of the hospital and the twentieth of the School. The Jubilee was celebrated on Monday 6 June when Her Majesty Queen Elizabeth II visited the site; a world map showing the countries of origin of all the 12,000 students who had attended the School in the past 20 years – from every country except Japan and Nicaragua – was a major exhibit and thereafter was placed on the wall of the School Secretary's office (and became Miss O'Driscoll's most effective placator for those waiting to see the Dean). The next day distinguished visitors were shown round, while on the third day the School and Hospital were open to the public. The Duke of Edinburgh made a private visit on 7 December to see research in progress and 'talk to the workers'. As a result of all this the Hammersmith Hospital and Postgraduate Medical School Association (known as the Hammersmith Postgraduate Association) was formed and held an open day on 4 July 1956. There were 500 members and in the evening a dinner was held at the Royal College of Surgeons. The Association flourished for the next 20 years, but with the passage of time fewer 'old boys' attended and it ceased to exist in its original form.

In quick succession, capital works followed in 1957 (new operating theatres, extension to the central stores, upgrading of wards, day rooms, staff quarters, records office, piped oxygen, and so on) until 1961. The complaints for which patients were admitted to hospital were very different after 1951. The need for beds declined, to be superseded by the need for a bigger out-patient department, more operating theatres, better laboratories and a larger X-ray department. As hospital treatment became more efficient and effective more patients came to hospital but there was no room to house them. By 1960 it was no longer government policy to have more hospital beds but new and better hospitals, and all political parties referred to hospital buildings in their manifestos for the 1959 General Election.

THE 1962 HOSPITAL PLAN

On 23 January 1962, Enoch Powell, Minister of Health in Macmillan's new government, submitted 'The Hospital Plan for England and Wales' for Parliament's approval.[67] Ninety new hospitals of 600 beds each were to be built, 134 to be remodelled substantially (which included Hammersmith) and 356 other major schemes were to be started by 1971. The cost of these schemes was expected to be £500 million. More than that, the expectation was that, by 1975, £700 million would provide 750 modern hospitals to replace the existing 2800 in England and Wales. It was a major and imaginative reorganization of the entire hospital service – and wildly optimistic in spite of agreement by the Treasury to long-term planning and investment in the Service.

The 1962 Plan had taken 2 years to prepare. There was a lack of surveyors, engineers and doctors capable of planning, so a team went to the U.S.A. to study the latest developments in hospital building: as a result, the Ministry of Health issued 'Hospital Building Notes', a series of diagrams and text as a guide for the future. A site of 30 acres was recommended for a 600-bed hospital, although this might be less in some urban areas. The general philosophy of The Plan was to determine the expected demand for health services then supply services to satisfy that demand. It was expected that the demand would depend on the number and composition of the population, the average incidence of disease and injuries, the type of treatment required and the most suitable method of providing it. It was not realized that failure to define accurately the demand was a central defect in the philosophy, and that a large group of doctors at the Hammersmith were working towards the different objective of creating new demands as a direct consequence of their own researches and developments on site.

Colonel W. Parkes, Chairman of the House Committee responsible to the Board of Governors of Hammersmith Hospital for the day-to-day management of affairs, wrote in the Annual Report for the Hospital 1961–1963: 'It is a matter of congratulation that provision has been made for the substantial extension of the Hospital in the near future and that work on the new Central Block will commence at an early date. We eagerly look forward to the time when the long years of planning bear fruit in the shape of modern buildings designed and equipped to enable this great Teaching Hospital to meet the needs of those it serves.' And so did everyone else! The Report included a photograph of what the new Hospital and School would look like by about 1971: the manipulated photograph bears a strong resemblance to the average U.S.A. City Hospital. The planned extra 400 new beds would bring the total complement to 850 beds. It was to cost £4.5 million and the University had agreed to provide an extra £800,000 for academic facilities. The future looked rosy.

The construction was to be carried out in two phases. Phase 1 was the construction of a basement, sub-basement, and ground floor on which there would be a modern out-patient department: the existing out-patient department was built in 1935, large enough for 20,000 patient-attendances a year but for the past 10 years had had to cope with over 100,000. Phase 2 would consist of two wards, each designed on the 'race-track' or double-corridor principle with beds on the periphery of the ward and ancillary accommodation in the middle – the central access core being at the right angle of the L for service and passenger lifts. Each floor was intended for a particular specialty. The top four floors would be of unusual design and ventilation so that both medical and surgical patients requiring special treatments (mainly immunological depressants for kidney and marrow grafts) could be nursed in sterile surroundings. Phase 1 was expected to start in the autumn of 1964 and Phase 2 to follow immediately.

In addition, an Investigation Block[68] of laboratories and examination rooms – the cost and use to be shared by the Hospital Board of Governors and the Postgraduate Medical School – was to be joined to the eastern side of the Central Ward Block and linked by bridges to the School's Laboratory Block. Architects were engaged and a great many people spent a great deal of time designing buildings that bore little relationship to reality. Unemployment at 878,356 was the highest since 1947, Britain had had continuous night frosts from 22 December 1962 to 6 March 1963, the Profumo affair had heralded the end of Macmillan as Prime Minister, and money was tight. In October 1964 Harold Wilson was elected Prime Minister for the Labour Party with a majority of five in the House of Commons, and Hammersmith Hospital became uneasy about its future rebuilding plans.

A new boiler house was constructed in the north-east corner of the site to provide energy for the new Hospital, School and Medical Research Council buildings. The new School Laboratory Block, as it was then called, had already begun and this was expected to be finished before hospital building started. The Chairman of The Governors, Sir Desmond Morton, wrote the foreword to the 1964–65 Annual Report. The vision of a new hospital was receding: 'deferred' was the term used. His consolation lay in a new supervoltage (a cobalt and linear accelerator) Radiotherapy Unit, begun in 1964, which was likely to be in use towards the end of the year: with Hospital and School both constructing major buildings on each side of the Wolfson Institute, in an overcrowded site, this was quite an achievement!

The National Hospital Rebuilding plan of 1962 was based on 3.8% growth in the national economy for the next 6 years: in fact, growth was reduced to 2% by 1964. Harold Wilson had the vision of a new industrial efficiency, to be attained through technical advance and economic and political planning. He was enchanted by the new technology, and believed that the sixties would complement the forties (when the Attlee government had nationalized half a dozen industries, and the Hammersmith Hospital). Socialists of the older generation had laid the foundation of the Welfare State; Socialists of the next generation, better at economics and more alive to business needs, would make it work. The State would provide money and direction for industrial output to grow, with modern inventions and modern management techniques.

The General Election in March 1966 gave the Labour Party a 97-seat majority in Parliament, and a clear vote for the 'white hot technological revolution', but on 27 July there was a 6 months freeze on prices, wages and salaries, and the economy staggered to a halt. The new School of 1966 – for that is what the Central Laboratory Block really was, later to be called the Commonwealth Building in recognition of its new role and former donors – was born in the same troubled financial poverty as the original of 1935. The 31 years difference in age spanned miracles in medicine but no change in its status, continually short of money, continually bursting with new ideas. Major hospital building, as far as Hammersmith was concerned, was over. From now on 'expansion' would be by 'in-filling' between existing buildings.

The opening of the new Medical School, known appropriately as the Commonwealth Building because that was where the money to build it had come from, provided 12 floors of 11,000 m^2 total, an increase of five times the 1935 School. Everyone was delighted. The fact that the School now had the amount of accommodation it should have had in the first place, and it thought it needed, and had raised the money for it by individual effort, was a matter of rejoicing.

ROYAL

On 26 October 1966 Roy Jenkins the Home Secretary wrote to Lord Stamp: 'I am glad to inform you that, on my recommendation, the Queen has approved that the Postgraduate Medical School of London shall in future be known as the "Royal Postgraduate Medical School" '. There followed much correspondence to have the new charter incorporated, and particularly to make sure that the school was not now named 'The Royal . . .': that so much paper could be generated by the definite article was surprising, but the Dean did not want it and the office of the Lord Chancellor did. On 28 July 1967 the Queen in Council at the Court at Buckingham Palace approved the petition submitted, thus completing a process which had started 3 years earlier.

The Dean convened an open day, a *conversazione* in November, to show 1000 guests the various departments now housed in the new building, what they do, how they work and something of their past achievements. It was the chance to show generous benefactors, colleagues and friends what the Hammersmith was all about and to say 'thank you' in public. But there was too much to see. It was the first time that individual departments had opened their doors wide to others: no member of staff had appreciated just how much work was going on under his nose, and by popular request the many exhibitions were retained for 3 weeks simply to allow 'in-house' appreciation. The Photographic Department had supplied over 700 full-plate and poster-size pictures and every department had exhibition stands demonstrating work done, sometimes work to be done, but all of interest if somewhat amateurish in display. The Annual Report recorded: 'Many people working here together with their families, were able, often for the first time, to take the opportunity of seeing what goes on at Hammersmith. Some of the local schools sent large groups of pupils'. Many pupils were knowledgeable of the research techniques used and, surprisingly, of Hammersmith's past achievements such as the heart-lung machine, kidney transplants, the radium bomb.

The people of Canada donated an Eskimo sculpture in green soap-stone, the largest in the U.K., which was mounted in the south-east corner of the entrance hall of the new building: it was of an Eskimo woman fishing at a hole in the ice with a salmon at her feet, and a papoose on her back holding a snow goose. Joseph Collier generously donated £50,000 for a new building for cardiovascular research, constructed by Bovis Ltd in the courtyard of L block (the site of the library hut in 1947 and commonly known as the Dean's garden because it contained a gold-fish pond and three metres square of paving), and opened officially by the Rt Hon. Anthony Crosland, Secretary of State for Education and Science. This housed Shillingford's M.R.C. Cardio-Vascular Unit, while new laboratories of the roof of L block accommodated Booth's M.R.C. research group on malabsorption.

On 14 April 1967 Sir George Godber,[69] Chief Medical Officer of the Ministry of Health (and a good friend of the School) formally opened the Computer Centre on the third floor of the Commonwealth Building: a unit operated jointly by the School and Elliott Medical Automation who had provided the digital computer at a cost of £60,000 (the National Research Development Corporation gave generous financial assistance). In the same month the Wellcome Unit of Endocrinology (Fraser and MacIntyre) was set up by a grant of £100,000: Fraser was to take care of the clinical side and MacIntyre of the endocrine chemistry (he was later to be a prime mover in the story of the discovery of calcitonin and its relation to medullary cancer of the thyroid). The unit was accommodated on the sixth floor.

The old lecture theatre in South Corridor (outside of which rests the plaque commemorating the laying of the foundation stone of the School by Neville Chamberlain) modernized by a grant from the M.P. Shah Foundation to hold 100 attenders with up-to-date visual aids and electronic stethoscopes (so that 100 could hear the heart beat of a single patient simultaneously), was opened by His Excellency the High Commissioner for India on 26 November 1968. A bridge joining the Experimental Surgical Laboratories and the ninth floor of the new medical school, not level but effective, and hoisted into position on a blustery Sunday morning – it was 72 feet long and 115 feet above ground level – was officially opened as the 'Aird Bridge' by Sir Hedley Atkins, President of the Royal College of Surgeons, on 19 June 1969. It linked two important buildings, but many refused for emotional reasons to use it.

THE TODD REPORT OF 1968

The Todd Report (the Royal Commission on Medical Education 1965–1968) was published[70] and formally acknowledged, but 'it would be true to say that most of us view it with mixed feelings'. It contained no acknowledgement of the contribution to medical education by the British Postgraduate Federation, or by Hammersmith, its largest institute. 'The Report offers no clear plan for us in the future and, indeed, shows a remarkable neglect of the pattern of training to which we try to expose our graduates: research, teaching and exemplary clinical care.' That was how the Dean, Selwyn Taylor, dismissed it. Certainly the Todd Report of 1968 was never openly debated, nor did it take note in its manpower recommendations of many relevant changes of that time: the falling birth rate, the decline in professional medical emigration from Britain, the increase in the number of women students, the effect of inflation and the slowing down of Government money being invested in medicine. The report was discussed at Hammersmith, in the large Wolfson lecture theatre, by 100 academic staff and others: no decision was made, but it was a good debate and demonstrated the difference between faith and practicalities.

Finally, in January 1969 a research appeal was launched to solve the 'financial stringency' to which the universities had been subjected. The target was £700,000 and by June had reached £118,000, but it never attained the total envisaged for one simple reason: in everyday language people will give money for equipment or a building (something tangible), not for their use, maintenance, development or even their product; a sad reflection on human nature which every generation has to learn anew.

10

Growth: Staff (1945–1966)

The staffing of the School has always differed from that of other medical schools. In 1935 four University Professors and four Readers were appointed: these were the only permanent employees of the University, even though there had been the suggestion, at preliminary discussions on the founding of the School, that the Professors should be appointed for 5 years in the first instance, but this had been over-ruled. Within 10 years all Readers had left to become Professors. Next in line were First Assistants, posts held for 2 years and paid at a salary of £300 a year, just an eighth of the rate for a Professor (interestingly, 50 years later the equivalent post holder often earned more than a Professor).

There were four First Assistants in the Department of Medicine: G. H. Jennings (General Medicine), J. G. Scadding (Respiratory), P. H. Wood (Cardiovascular), J. F. Brock (Metabolism); four in Surgery: A. J. Watson (Orthopaedics and Fractures), A. L. Light (Genitourinary), G. V. Feggetter (Gastroenterology), R. H. Franklin (General); two in Obstetrics and Gynaecology, G. W. Theobald and Maeve Kenny; four in Pathology: Janet Vaughan (Clinical Pathology), F. D. Johnstone (Bacteriology), G. A. D. Haslewood (Pathological Chemistry), C. V. Harrison (Morbid Anatomy).

Finally there were House Physicians and House Surgeons who were usually selected from those attending courses at the Hammersmith, presumably the brightest and keenest. They were unpaid, which was the usual practice in London voluntary hospitals (and the practice persisted in some until 1948!) in the same way that visiting consultants were not paid except for teaching. The consultant earned money from his private practice and used the good name of the voluntary hospital to further his reputation as well as relying on the referral of patients by his ex-students: the houseman earned pocket money by doing evening locums for general practitioners. Housemen did, of course, receive free board and lodgings: it was the reputation of the 'board' as much as that of the 'chief' that attracted trainees to a particular hospital. In 1937 it was decided that 'Hammersmith housemen should be paid 100 guineas a year' (105 pounds).

The Consultants visited the School once a week and at other times to 'see cases at the request of the Director'. It was not part of their duties to give instruction to students, but 'in some cases they have developed moderate-sized out-patient clinics' (and so presumed safe to teach some students, but not paid for that). Those appointed in the first year were: R. T. Brain (Dermatology), Laming Evans (Orthopaedics – note that Orthopaedics did not automatically include fractures at this time), Purdon Martin (Neurology), Aubrey Lewis (Psychology), A. A. Moncrief (Paediatrics, and later to become the first Professor of Paediatrics at the Institute of Child Health), R. C. Davenport (Ophthalmology) and Sydney Scott (Otolaryngology). The audited accounts for 1936 showed an expenditure of £1147 for this service (or £163 per annum per consultant). In addition, each of the three clinical Departments had a Senior Assistant Medical Officer, appointed and paid for by the London County Council.

The staff were further divided into 'A' and 'B' staff. The 'A' staff were whole-time and permanently appointed to the School (Professors and Readers appointed by the University of London). The 'B' staff included members of the medical profession invited from time to time to take part in the teaching activities of the School. They were 'occasional teachers' and in 1936 their salaries totalled £375/18/0. More importantly, their services were used in four ways. First, as an acknowledged authority on some branch of medicine, they were invited to deliver a course of lectures: these were publicized widely in London and the titles recorded in the Annual Report of the School. Second, courses of lectures covering recent advances were organized, each being given by a selected lecturer. Third, many were employed mainly in Intensive Courses for general practitioners, usually teachers whose writings were already familiar to them. Fourth, two leading teachers of medicine would take charge of a ward and give two clinics a week for limited periods: for example Lord Horder came from 22 September to 18 December 1935, and Sir Arthur Hall from 3 May to 15 July 1936.

There were also Voluntary Assistants who came, unpaid and probably carefully selected, for 6–12 months helping with routine work in a Department and carrying out some investigations on their own. Finally, Demonstrators of Clinical Medicine were employed to help supervise students' work: they attended for three half-days a week, and were often recipients of Medical Research Council grants for specific research projects but who needed access to clinical material.

In 1937 it was agreed that the School should take one house physician and one house surgeon each from the Royal Navy and the Army, and from the Indian Medical Service, to remain on the wards for 10 weeks twice yearly. These doctors were of good calibre and welcomed: the practice continued into the late seventies. Major-General Drew R.A.M.C. (and one of the above) was to state later that the Hammersmith and the Army benefited: during the 1939–1945 war the School conducted 72 special war courses which were attended by 3700 officers from British, American, Canadian and other forces and almost certainly had the effect of spreading the School's reputation abroad because the officers attending were able to see the quality of the research work in progress and its implication for teaching.

STAFF TITLES

When the creation of a Federation of Institutes seemed likely the School reorganized the titles of the teaching staff and adjusted their salaries to fit in with their new status; clerical and technical staff were allowed 24 working days holiday in the year and their salary rates transferred to the University scale. The term First Assistant (a title to continue at the University of Oxford until the mid-seventies when it was changed to Clinical Reader, but without tenure) became Lecturer: Lecturer at other medical schools meant non-consultant and in the National Health Service after 1948 was the equivalent of Senior Registrar. At the Postgraduate Medical School of London all Lecturers were, in fact and without question, consultants and invariably held an honorary consultant appointment within the N.H.S. at the Hospital; the term Senior Lecturer was an honour reserved for part-time senior members of staff.

The title Lecturer did not bring job security in the same way that it did for consultants in the N.H.S.; it did not even bring equality of pay until 1953! On the contrary, a Lecturer's contract was for 1 year renewable annually, dependent on 'productivity', and his salary was at the non-medical University rate. On 9 March 1961 the University Grants Committee made its quinquennial visitation spending a whole day at the School, and instead of looking at buildings, talked to all grades of staff group-by-group. Sir John Wolfenden,[71] later to become Chairman, listened to 18 irate and vocal full-time Lecturers: it was a frank and open discussion. They did not complain of overwork, underpay, or lack of security, but that 1 year was insufficient time in which to complete a research project. As a result the appointment was extended to 5 years! Of those 18, 10 became Professors within a decade.

THE METHOD OF APPOINTMENTS

Another area of contention lay in the methods by which appointments were made in the School. Appointees were vetted closely, assessed on the quality and originality of their work, and selected almost entirely on merit. The appointment was made by consensus directed by one person: the idea that a committee could do the job better was discounted by common experience. Nearly all staff were active researchers before coming to the Hammersmith, some were seconded with research scholarships. But in 1948 when the expected provisions of the N.H.S. became known the School attempted to revise its method of making appointments. An Appointments Advisory Committee was instituted on which there were representatives of the University, of the Royal Colleges, and of the School. The innovation proved to be a little cumbersome and time-consuming, but was superseded by the N.H.S. Act regulations: the Dean wrote: 'it is hoped that these will not fulfil the rather gloomy anticipations foreshadowed by the School Appointments Committee'. In defence of this attitude of suspicion, it should be pointed out that over 30 years later no commercial company in the U.K. appoints its top executives in the manner recommended in 1948: 'head hunting' is still the quickest and most effective way to obtain the person required. Moreover, no commercial company, now or in 1948, allowed outsiders to choose their appointee. Democracy, or at least this form fabricated for the N.H.S., was thought by School staff unlikely to select the outstanding person. The job of a committee, even an appointments committee, is to reach a compromise; a compromise candidate was the last thing that the Hammersmith could afford, and this was borne out by events in 1978 when N.H.S. Consultants were brought in to fill gaps in clinical services.

It would, however, be untrue to pretend that the Hammersmith did not resist the N.H.S. pressures, and successfully, until about the mid-sixties. The technique was to accept a research fellow, paid for by a reputable grant-giving body (the Medical Research Council, Nuffield Foundation, Wellcome Trust), whose expertise fitted into the general direction of the School's work, to claim honorary consultant status from the Hospital for the clinical work being done free for the N.H.S., and at the end of the term of grant-support (usually 3 years but extendable for much longer terms) to appoint that person to a University post. In this way it was possible to avoid the embarrassment of having to advertise the post to fill a gap in the hospital service and then be landed with a non-research and ineffective member of the School's staff: other hospitals were welcome to take pot-luck, not Hammersmith. The system proved curiously effective but was destroyed when the University was no longer able to pay new salaries, yet the N.H.S. could. The effect of this loss of flexibility and freedom of choice has still to be assessed.

Almost as a replacement for the N.H.S. system of appointments Hammersmith created personal chairs. Lewis and Maude[72] had commented that 'to be a professional man or woman today is to live with uncertainty', and Hammersmith emphasized this by annual reviews of its Lecturers. What it did not do, and so far has not done, was to bow to outside pressures to grant tenure (that is the appointment of university teachers to retiring age on contracts that cannot

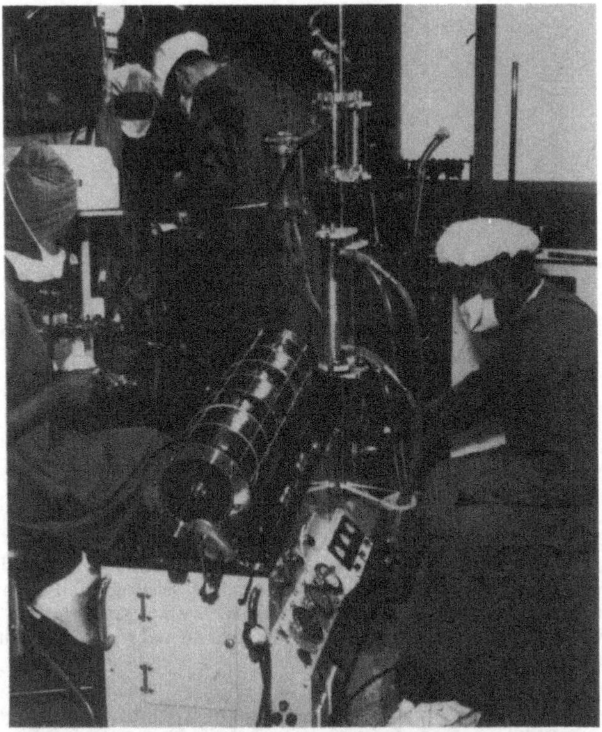

Figure 31 The heart–lung machine in use in the operating theatre in 1961

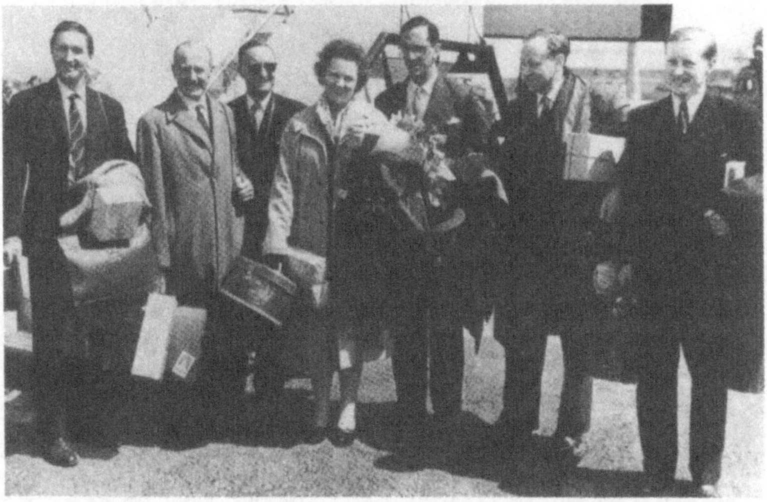

Figure 32 The heart–lung team which sailed for Russia, 23 April 1959. Left to right: Melrose (inventor of the artificial lung), Robson (chief technician), Bentall (cardiac surgeon), Bowtle (theatre sister), Beard (anaesthetist), Cleland (cardiac surgeon), Holman (cardiac physician). The *Daily Telegraph* newspaper of 24 April 1959 quoted Bill Cleland as saying, 'we put a yellow rose on top of the machine for every operation'

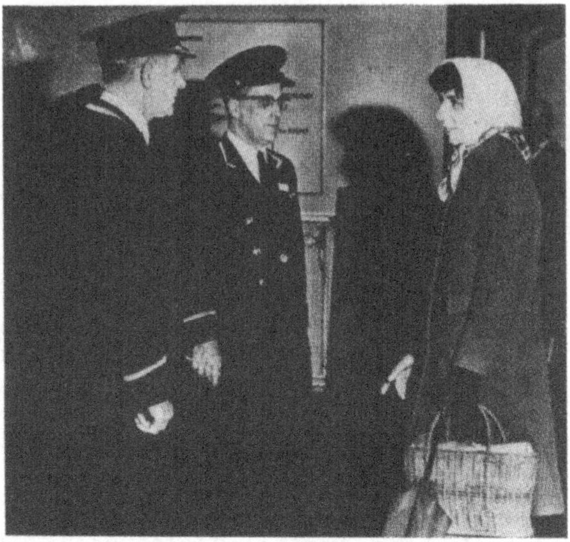

Figure 33 *c.* 1967. The Hospital Hall Porters. Mr James (retired 1968) and Mr House (retired 1971) talking to a visitor in the entrance hall of the Hospital. Both men were well-known by patients, staff and visitors for the service they gave (a total of 75 years): they wore dark green long coats piped with gold braid and peaked caps with (the L.C.C. crest) badges

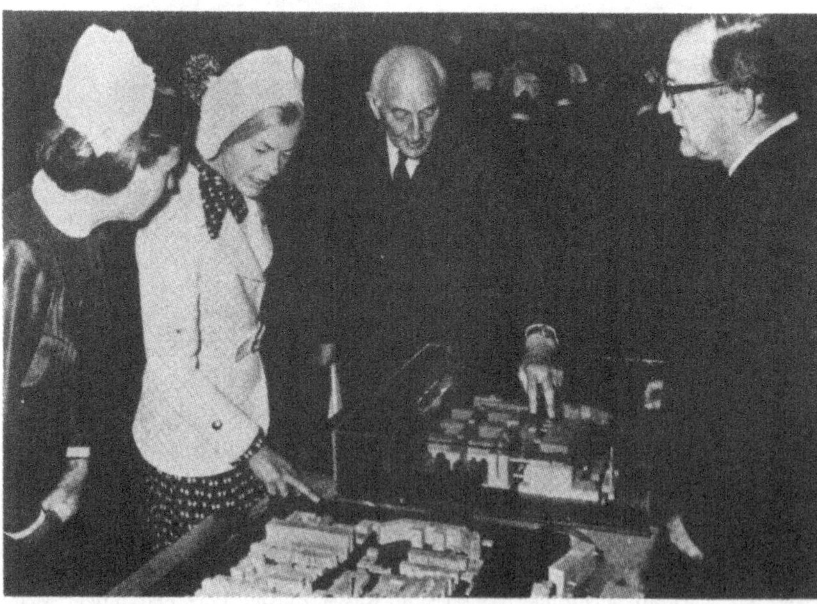

Figure 34 H.R.H. The Duchess of Kent inspecting models of the future hospital, during the Nurses' Prizegiving Day in 1971. Left to right: Miss Fraser-Gamble (Matron), H.R.H., Lord Cottesloe (Chairman, Board of Governors of the Hospital), Captain Dunlop R.N. Retd. (Developments Manager)

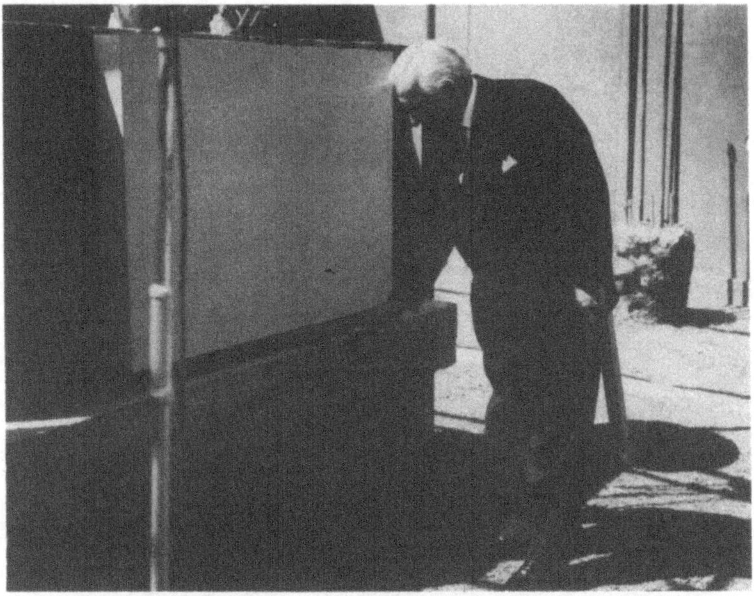

Figure 35 2 June 1959. Sir Isaac Wolfson laying the foundation stone of the Wolfson Institute

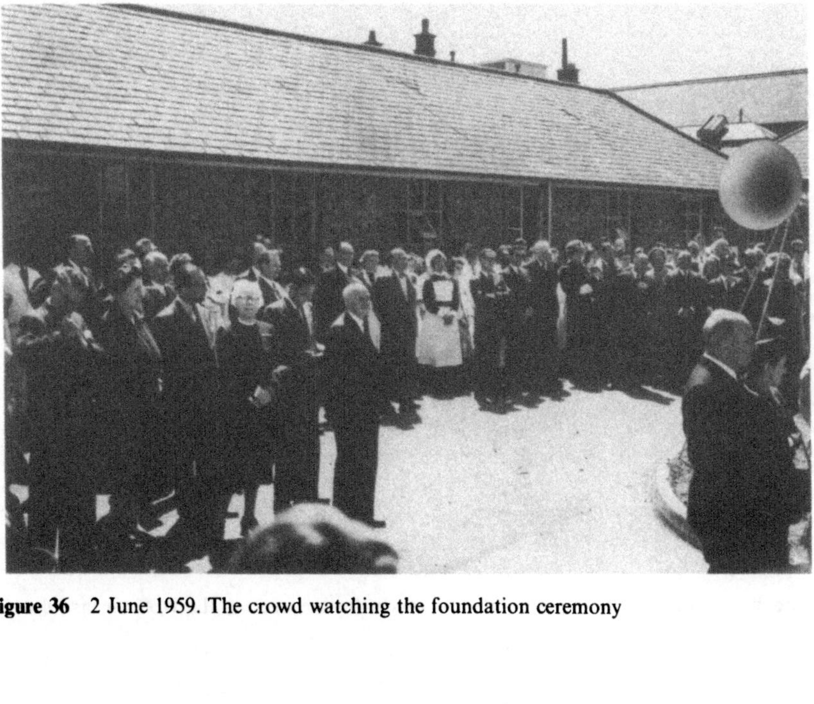

Figure 36 2 June 1959. The crowd watching the foundation ceremony

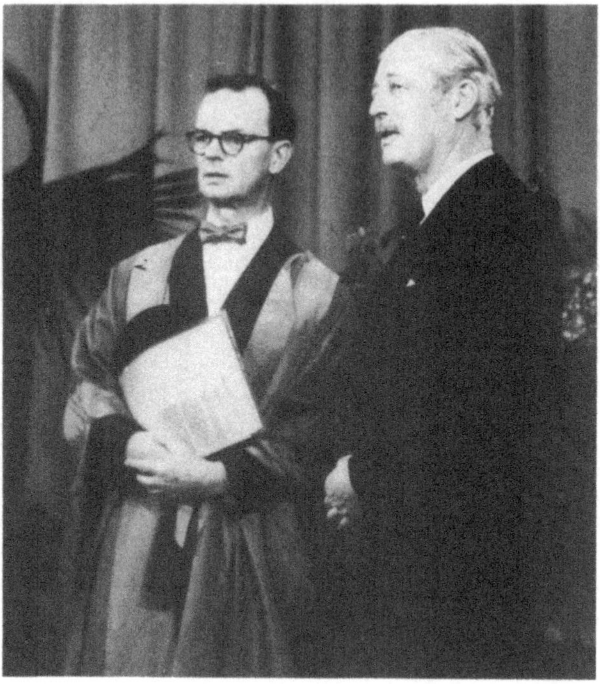

Figure 37 3 May 1961. The Dean (Dr Charles Newman) and the Prime Minister (Sir Harold Macmillan) when the latter officially opened the Wolfson Institute

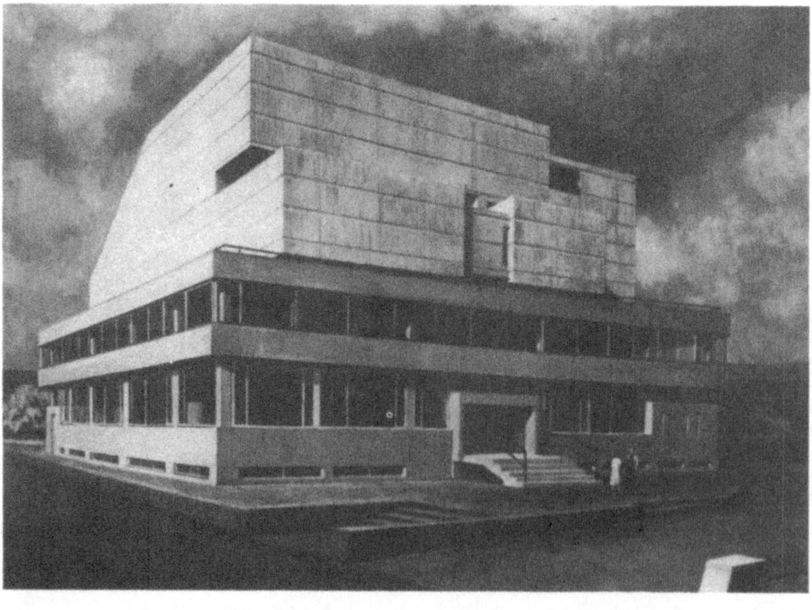

Figure 38 Artist's impression (accurate too, except for the trees) of the Wolfson Institute

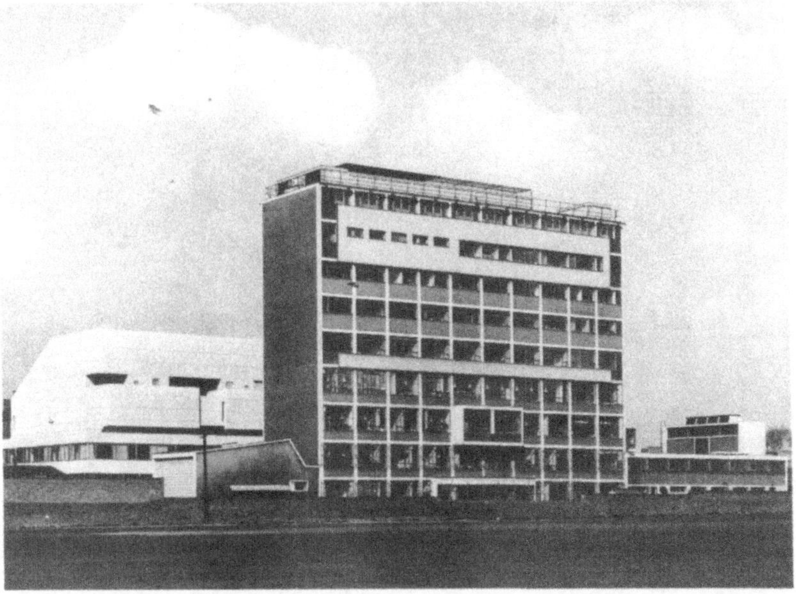

Figure 39 *c*. 1962. View from the playing fields of St Clement Danes School of the Wolfson Institute (white) and the Surgical Research Laboratories (top four floors added to the M.R.C. Cyclotron Building)

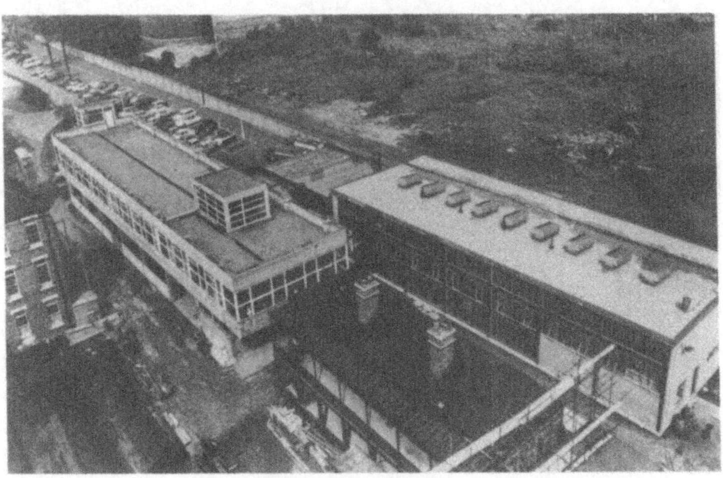

Figure 40 1963. The new oil-fired boiler-house (right), new hospital workshops for plumbers, carpenters, electricians (centre), recently constructed car park (top left) and recently demolished army recruiting huts on the Scrubs (top right)

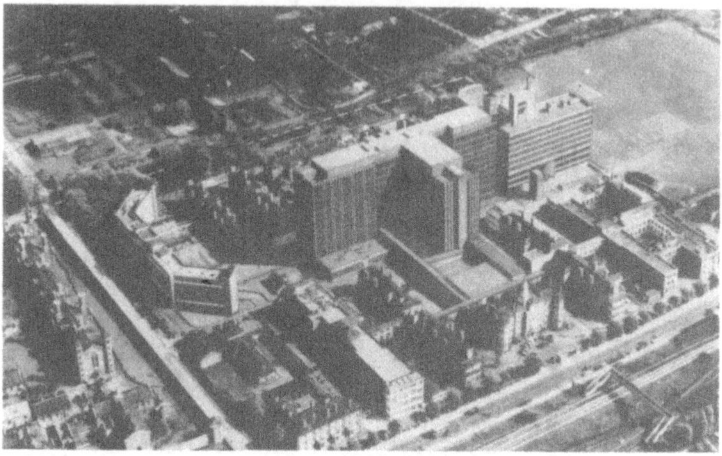

Figure 41 The planners' dream: aerial view of what the new hospital would look like as envisaged in 1961

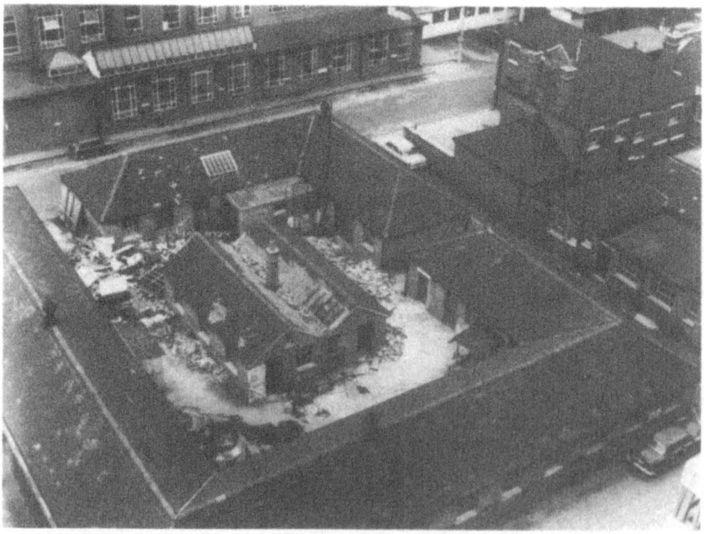

Figure 42 The building of the new medical school, December 1962. The M.R.C. workshops being demolished and (centre) the labour yard of the old workhouse (this meant hard labour): above, the School Pathology Department

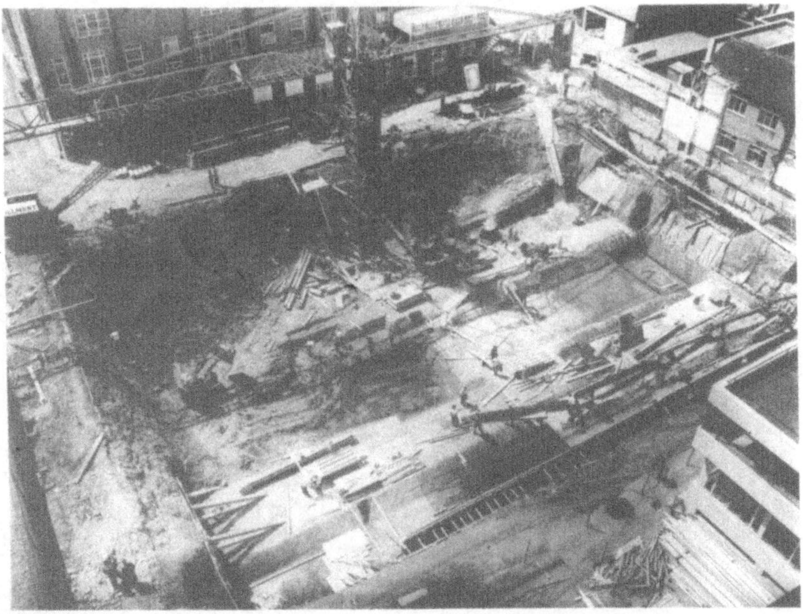

Figure 43 July 1963. The 'hole'. Note, bottom right, the Wolfson Institute and the shoring only in front of that building

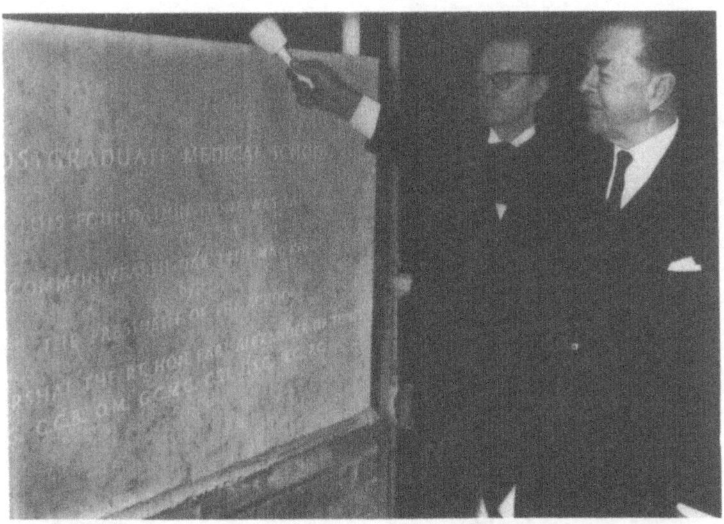

Figure 44 24 May 1963. Earl Alexander of Tunis (President of the School) lays the foundation stone of the Commonwealth Building with the Dean (Dr Charles Newman) watching

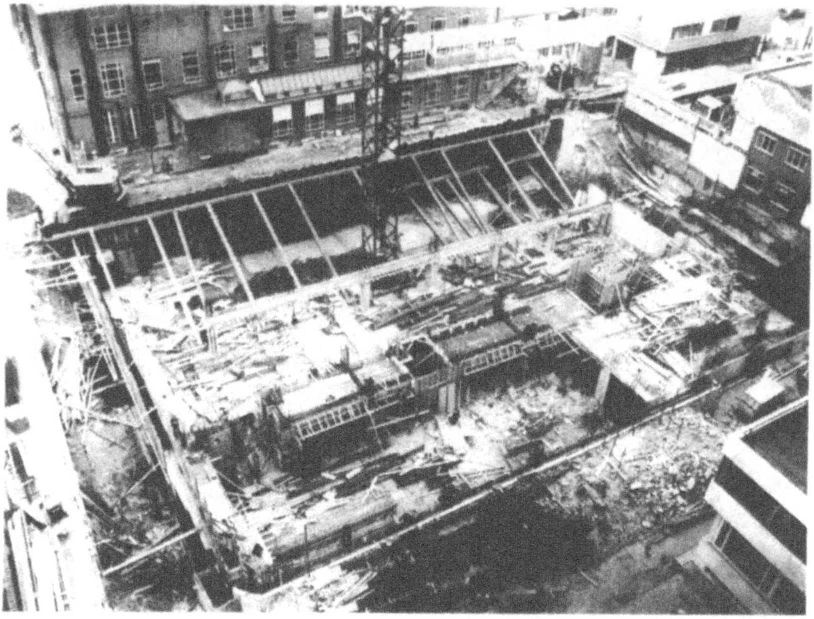

Figure 45 October 1963. The 'hole' with foundations and sub-basement of the Commonwealth Building nearly complete. Note the extensive shoring of the sides

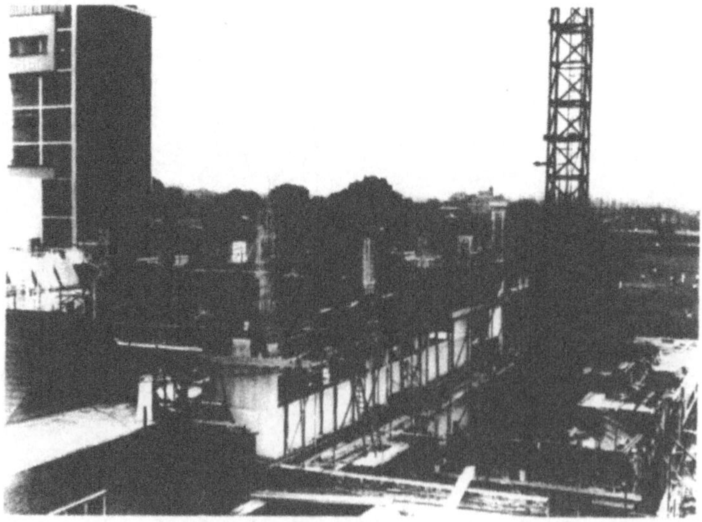

Figure 46 June 1964. Ground floor completed

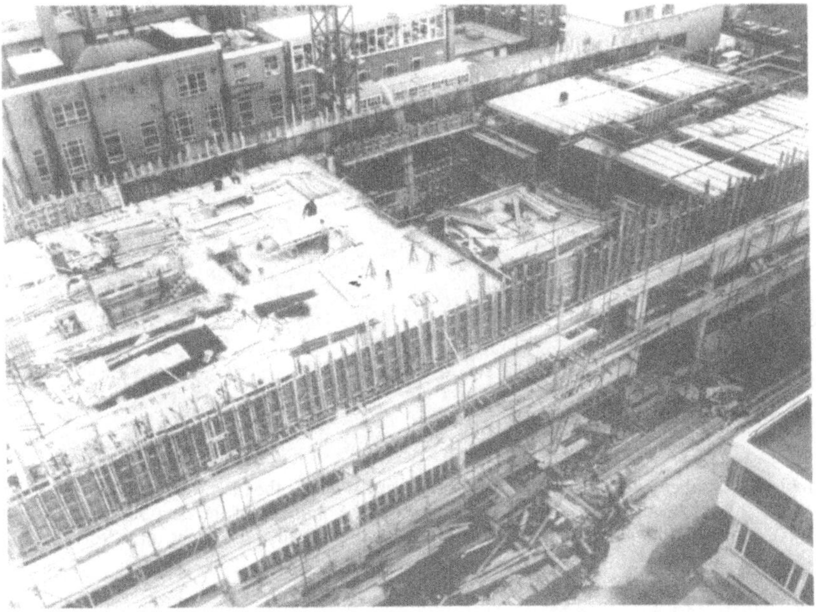

Figure 47 July 1964. Progress.

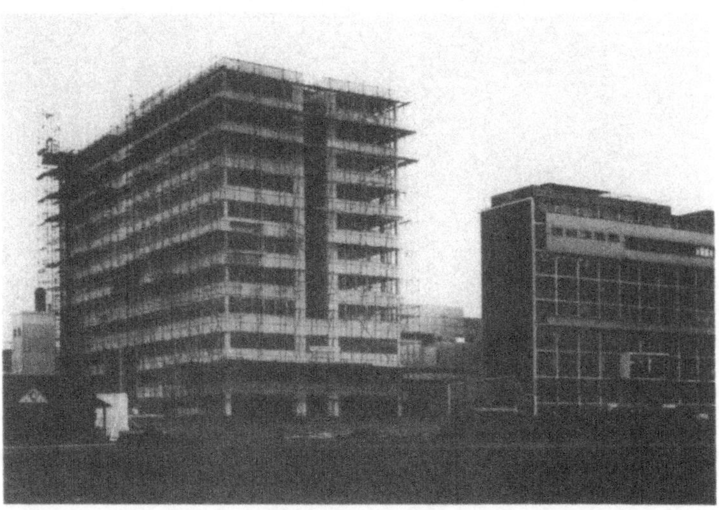

Figure 48 July 1965. The new Medical School nearing completion.

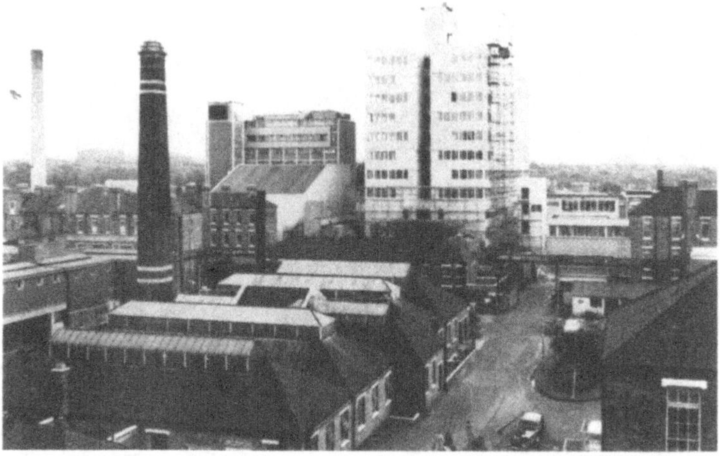

Figure 49 October 1965. The School from a different angle. In the foreground are the old boiler houses, laundry, linen room. Seen left is the chimney of the new boiler house and centre the two chimneys of the old; note the lagged water pipes on pylons

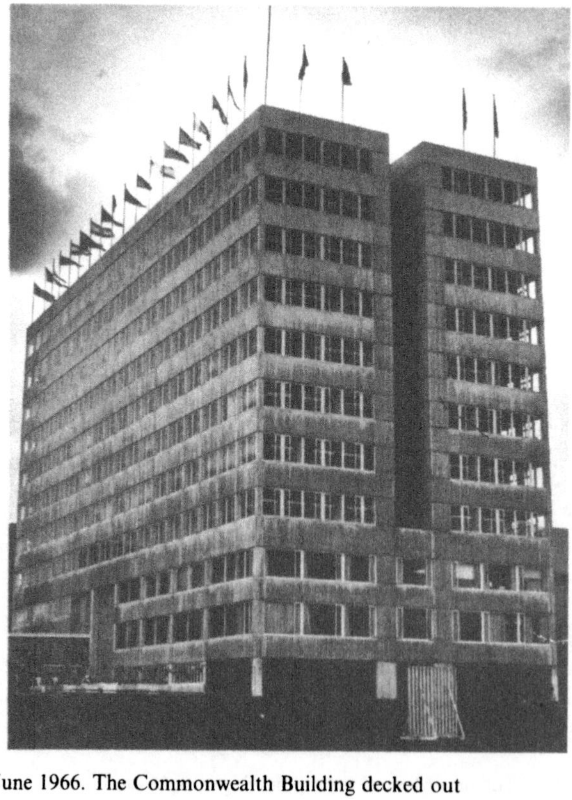

Figure 50 6 June 1966. The Commonwealth Building decked out

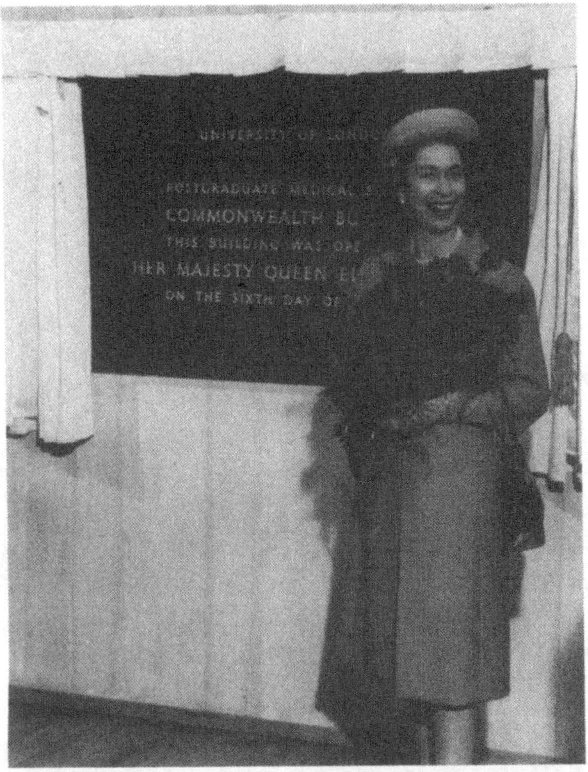

Figure 51 6 June 1966. H.M. Queen Elizabeth standing beside the commemorative plaque she had just unveiled

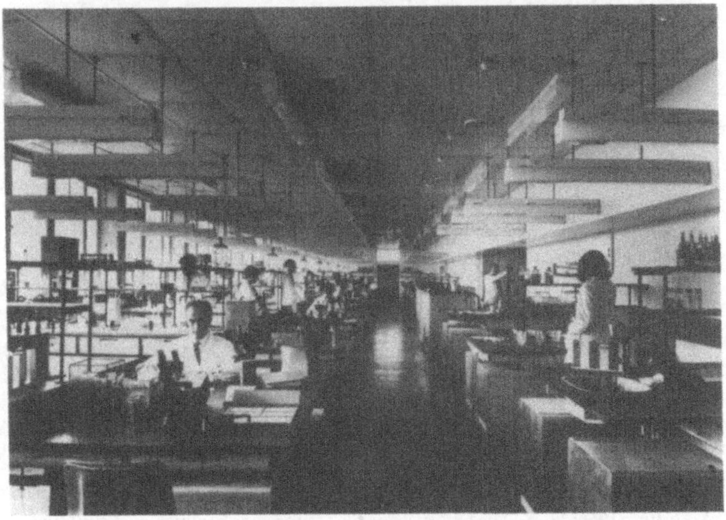

Figure 52 6 June 1966. The new laboratories for the D.C.P. Course waiting for the Royal visit

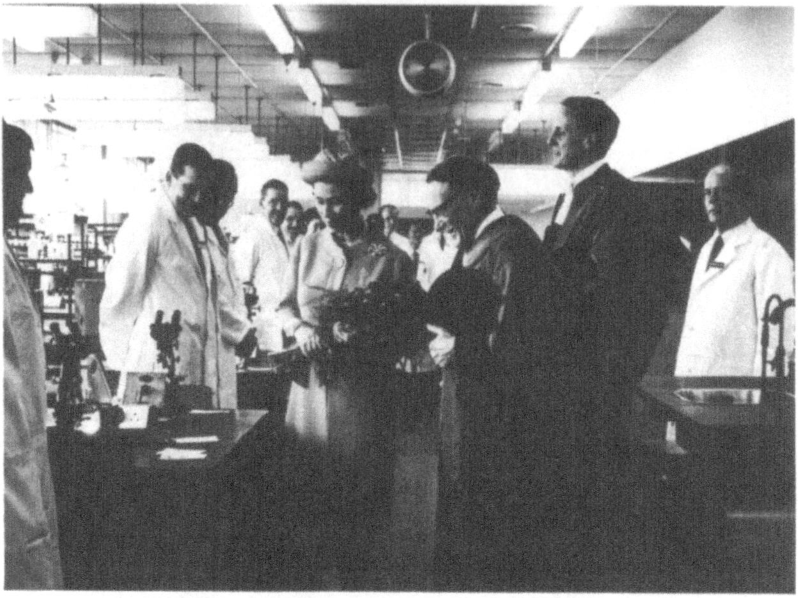

Figure 53 6 June 1966. H.M. The Queen inspecting the laboratory. In the centre is Professor Harrison and to the right the Dean (Mr Selwyn Taylor)

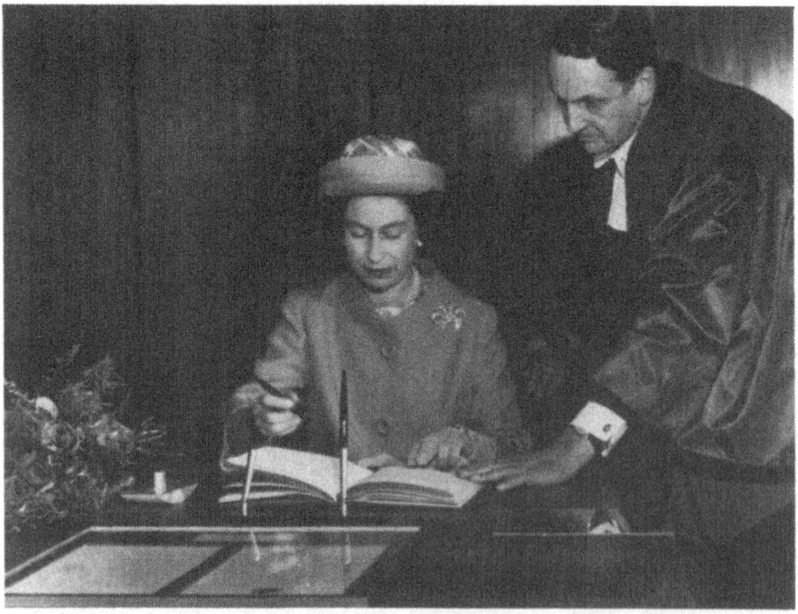

Figure 54 6 June 1966. H.M. The Queen signs the visitors book, which also contained the 1935 signature of her grandfather, King George V, and the Dean, Mr Selwyn Taylor

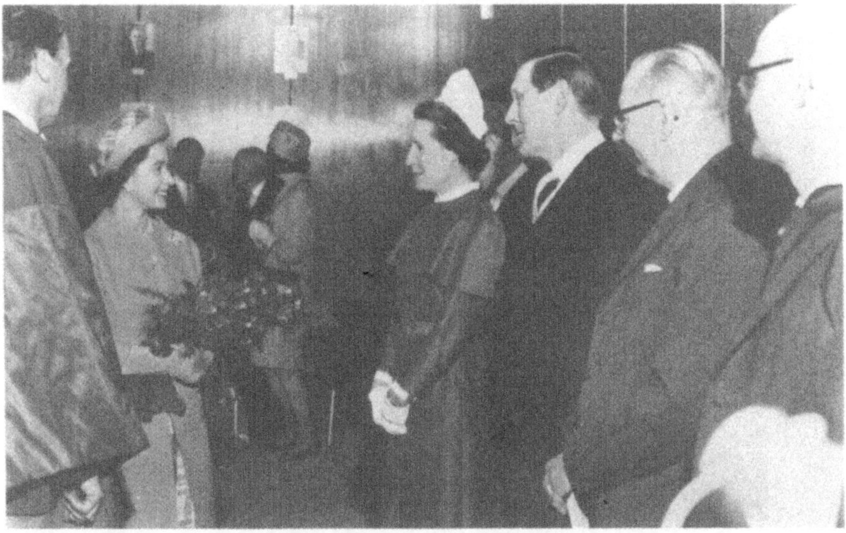

Figure 55 6 June 1966. H.M. Queen Elizabeth II talking to staff in the Board Room of the Commonwealth Building. Left to right: Taylor (Dean), H.M., Miss Fraser-Gamble (Matron of the Hospital), Mackay (Medical Superintendent of the Hospital), Barnes (School Accountant), Vellacott (School Secretary). Note photographs on the 'Wall of fame': Grey Turner, left, and Ian Aird, centre

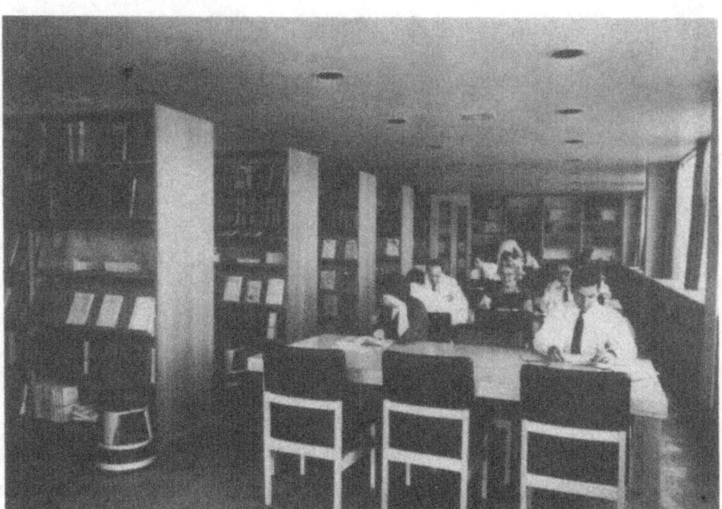

Figure 56 *c.* 1967. One side of the Wellcome Library looking towards the issue desk. The lady in the centre is Miss Dorothy Atkins, the chief librarian for 20 years

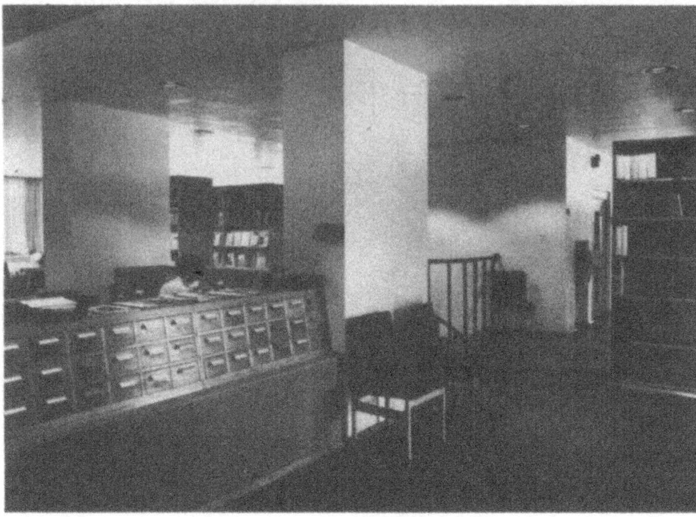

Figure 57 Issue desk and author/subject index of the Wellcome Library. The rails of the circular staircase leading to the floor below (stock room and carousels for private study) can be seen centre

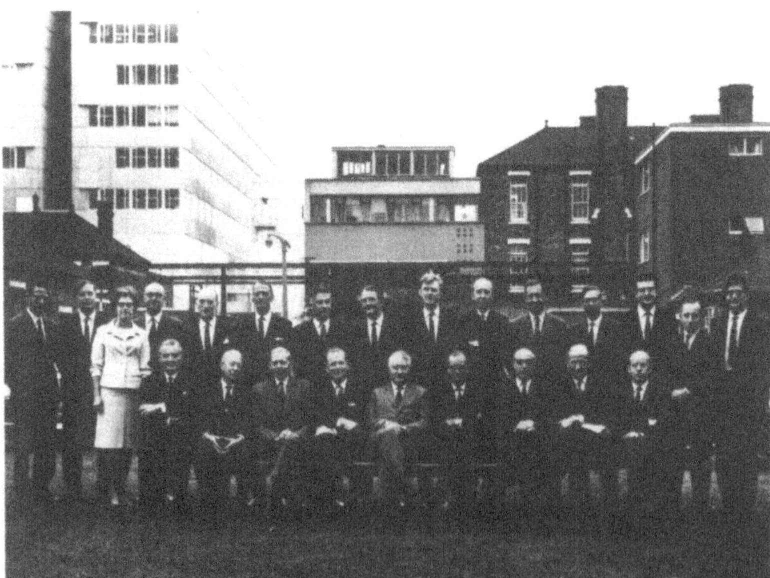

Figure 58 July 1966. The Department of Medicine at the time of the retirement of its head, Professor Sir John McMichael, consultant staff. Standing left to right: Poole, Brain, Oakley, Scott, Mounsey, Gilliland, Pallis, Booth, Dollery, Campbell, West, Joplin, Gabe, Davis, Seated: Shillingford, Cope, Goodwin, Fraser, McMichael, Bywaters, Scadding, Fletcher, Tizard

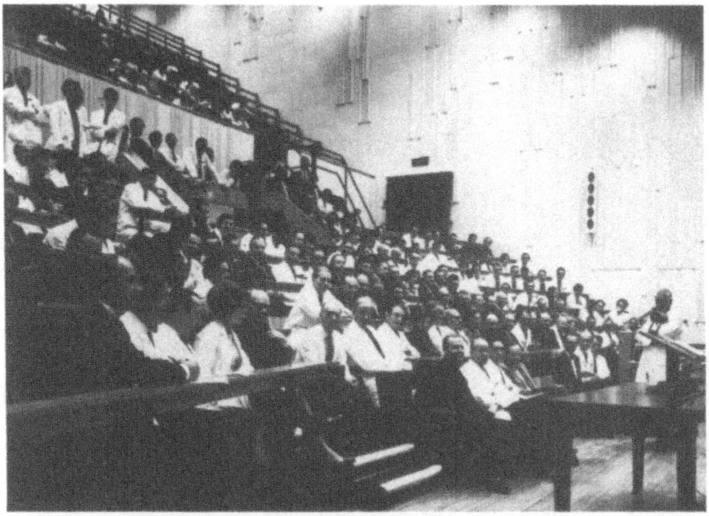

Figure 59 17 July 1966. Sir John McMichael's last staff-round and clinico-pathological conference in the large lecture theatre (The Stamp) of the Wolfson Institute, when many previous members of the Department of Medicine attended

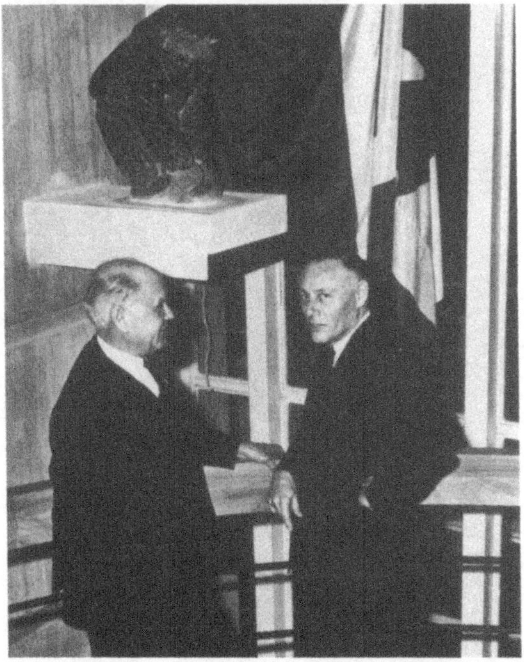

Figure 60 14 December 1967. Lord Stamp (Chairman of the School Building Appeal) and Heinz Blandford (School Treasurer) standing beneath the soapstone Eskimo sculpture presented by the Canadian Friends of the Postgraduate Medical School. It was unveiled by the wife of the School President, Lady Alexander of Tunis, in the presence of the High Commissioner of Canada

be broken by the employer) after only 3 years of probation and without a detailed review of the candidate's worthiness. It was not easy to resist, particularly when the Employment Acts of 1975 and 1976 tended to favour the individual on humanitarian grounds and not on those of efficiency and effectiveness at the job. The School retained the right of major review at the end of a 5-year appointment on the grounds that the protection and privileges that the University could confer should not be inherited nor automatically granted. If a Lecturer had performed well, at the end of 5 years he could be offered permanent employment as Senior Lecturer, or promoted to Reader: after another 5 years of productivity he might then be made a Professor in his subject, the holder of a personal chair which would lapse when he retired. In more recent years there has been a tendency to promote people to personal chairs more rapidly, which may have the adverse effect of stultifying their full potential.

11

Teaching

Medicine is one of the few professions that can trace its lineage back for more than 2000 uninterrupted years. The oath attributed to Hippocrates states: 'I will look upon him who shall have taught me this Art even as one of my parents. . . . I will impart this Art by precept,by lecture and by every mode of teaching, not only to my own sons, but to the sons of him who has taught me, and to disciples bound by covenant and oath, according to the Law of Medicine.' Indeed, for 2000 years medicine has been taught as an apprenticeship system by doctors who have never had any formal training for teaching.

Before the Second World War undergraduate teaching, in London and elsewhere, was a cosy affair mainly didactic and anecdotal. Established clinicians, the teachers, would demonstrate physical signs at ward rounds and out-patients clinics, give lectures, and ask questions. The students were expected to take notes, read standard textbooks (often written by the teacher) and give standard answers. The main aim was to pass examinations and qualify as a doctor licensed by the State to practise medicine. There was a curriculum and the General Medical Council was responsible in law for that.

POST-QUALIFICATON TEACHING

When Christopher Addison set up the Athlone Committee to look into Postgraduate Medicine in 1921 there was no mention of a curriculum, which is surprising in a way because Addison was a well qualified doctor – he was M.D., and F.R.C.S. and had trained at Bart's – but he was concerned with organization rather than content. The eminent men and women on that committee accepted the need for further education after qualification and had G.P.s mainly in mind, but had little idea of what postgraduate medicine meant. The Report of the Postgraduate Medical Education Committee of 1930 was no better: subcommittee B (Education) met on five occasions and concluded that no co-ordinated scheme of postgraduate instruction could be devised. Indeed on the third meeting the sixteen members had begun to relate teaching to the number of beds. Sir Thomas Horder, the Chairman and a consultant physician at St Bartholomew's Hospital, proposed the following plan for the Department of Medicine in the British Postgraduate Medical School: Professorial Unit, 40 beds, special courses on selected diseases (Diabetes, Lymphadenoma, Rheumatoid Arthritis) 20 beds each for three courses, 60 in all. Treatment of acute diseases, 40 beds. Special departments (neurological, paediatric, dermatology, cardiology), 20 each for four departments, 80 in all. The total beds for the Medical Department were to be 220.

It was pointed out that on this basis, if 220 was the minimum number of beds proper to be allocated to a Medical Department, the existing number of beds in the hospital (400) would be insufficient to enable a proper allocation to be made to the Surgical Department and to the Obstetric Department. There was a diagram of the organizational structure included and on this basis there was a recommendation for the London County Council to increase the bed complement to 600!

At the next meeting, and clearly not to be outdone, Professor Gask, the University representative and a surgeon, produced his own diagram of the organization for Surgery, but omitting the number of beds allocated to each division, which included a large department for Plastic Surgery (there were only two Plastic Surgeons in the whole of Britain at the time!), for Dental Surgery and for Orthopaedic Surgery – all of which smacked of First World War thinking. One member complained that there was no mention of psychotherapy, but there was agreement that 'facilities for research should be an essential part of the work in the School and Hospital' without clarifying what was meant.

Perhaps the nearest to a directive is to be found in the Royal Charter of 1931, 'to secure new and extended facilities for the further education of medical practitioners, with the objects of promoting the advancement of knowledge of the best methods of treatment of the sick, and the improved application of such methods. . . . To provide opportunity for the advancement of knowledge . . .'.

In the bound minute-book for 1934 of the Governing Body, of the British Postgraduate Medical School to be and dated 1 March 1934 but unsigned, there is a memorandum, possibly written by Professor Gask who had also served on the Chamberlain Committee of 1925, which reads: 'It is of the first importance that the teaching should be of a really high level – suitable for increasing the knowledge of the better grade of medical practitioners. The provision of "refresher courses" may well be regarded as an important item in the activities of the comprehensive postgraduate scheme. . . . Nevertheless this type of activity should not be allowed any chance of "swamping" the more advanced work which may be expected to appeal more particularly to graduates proposing to specialise in some one branch of medical practice. For these, courses of an essentially different character will be needed. The early stages of the School's work must be to a great extent provisional and on the experience then gained future courses will have to be designed.' That is exactly what did happen and what has happened ever since: the continuous evolution of medical teaching. 'It [the School] also may claim to have a distinctly international side since in countries like the United States of America and the Argentine (to mention only two) the desire for such an institution in London is constantly expressed. Great advantage can be expected to accrue to the School, and to the advance of Medicine. . . .'

Even today, 50 years later, there is no curriculum as such, the teachers do not hold teacher qualifications, and there is not a single member of staff with B.Ed. At the Hammersmith B.T.A. (Been to America, meaning the U.S.A. and Canada) is mandatory, B.Ed. an unnecessary embellishment neither required by the University nor favoured by the School. This situation is not entirely the result of tradition but of pragmatism. Appointments to the School were made on the basis of research ability rather than teaching prowess and there is no evidence that students ever suffered. In the University, Lecturers may not lecture, Readers may not read, Professors may not profess – the titles are almost meaningless in that context – but all must contribute to the advancement of knowledge, which is the prime purpose of a university.

Until the Postgraduate Medical School was founded, post-qualification courses were based largely on the undergraduate type of teaching. However, it was recognized that qualified general practitioners and undergraduates should not be taught in the same class: just whose ignorance might be exposed was never made clear, but the two were separated until the Todd Report of 1968 recommended union. For Hammersmith the problem was two-fold: how to design a technique of postgraduate education and who should teach the teachers? What was to be different from the traditional method of teaching medicine?

Before the war the School taught mainly general practitioners, from this country and from overseas. During the war it taught a variety of people: war courses for service personnel and, because of the disruption, some undergraduates. Teaching was to be based on the personal experience and knowledge of the teacher: the early war courses clearly were an embarrassment because the teaching both by staff and by outside lecturers was based on personal experience of the 1914–1918 war and therefore 20 years out of date. It was only in 1942 that the Dean could report that the majority of lectures were given by serving officers with up-to-date experience in the field.

Lectures played a major part. The Dean in his 1950 annual report complained that the Hammersmith did not have a lecture room that would hold as many as

80 students! Indeed the annual reports listed the names and subjects of those who came to lecture, almost as a prospectus for intending applicants, as evidence of the good things received by attenders. The lectures were factual, authoritative, always followed by dissecting questions: quite often the discussion was between the questioners, with the lecturer agreeing first with one side then the other. These occasions were a challenge to audience and lecturer: the challenge of who knew and understood the most. Curiously, in the same year J. A. Lauwerys,[74] Professor of Education in the University of London, thought that lectures were already out of date and overvalued as a form of teaching. He wrote: 'I have already indicated that educators and teachers, in general, continue to believe that the method has value, even though less than was thought. The tradition of university lecturing was established at a time when books were scarce and expensive. They are now cheap and numerous; and they contain all the facts that are needed. The lecture never was an instrument of great efficiency as regards teaching facts: its value was chiefly in inspiring zeal, in developing a liking and gift for criticism and analysis, in permitting some contact, albeit rather slight with persons of distinction.' Thirty years after these words were written the three lecture theatres in the Wolfson Institute at the School are in constant demand daily and heavily booked for many months ahead by outside bodies as well as by staff: the competition for space is fierce, and the death of the lecture seems further away than ever.

CLINICO-PATHOLOGICAL CONFERENCES

The clinico-pathological conference was adopted as a method of teaching right from the early days and is still popular; it is an example of the way an environment of teaching and investigation can catalyse new ideas and nurture them into major innovations. The origin must be credited to Richard Cabot at the Massachusetts General Hospital in the last century, who printed case histories of patients and the pathological findings for his students, and to Dr Wright at the same institute, who started weekly conferences: a significant contribution to medical education which found immediate favour at the Hammersmith as a source of entertainment and enlightenment. At its best here is how it worked. The history and clinical findings of a patient with an unusual problem (often a rare disease, because the Hammersmith tended to collect such), which had been fully investigated, were presented to an invited clinician for his expert opinion and before an audience of doctors who were equally unaware of the patient's diagnosis, treatment or outcome. The eminent visitor can ask for the results of a specific investigation and these are declared, demonstrated, and explained by a senior member of the discipline concerned. These experts, on the basis of their findings, offer their own diagnosis which is compared with that made by the doctor in charge of the patient, usually the presenter, and discussed by the eminent visitor. Finally, the pathologist presents and explains his findings, which may or may not complete the story.

It is a game of highly educated and astute guesswork in which the pathologist alone may know the answer. It is detective work at its best, where previous experience, scholarship, and the powers of deduction all play a part: sometimes it is salutary to learn that there are not enough clues by which to reach an acceptable conclusion. The method, however, is invaluable in teaching the mental processes that are involved in the making of a diagnosis, it sharpens and refreshes the instinct of an experienced doctor, and keeps everyone on their toes. From time to time an edited series – which of necessity shortens the duration and changes the language from spoken to written English, as well as omitting some very witty remarks from the floor – have been published in the *British Medical Journal* from 1952 onwards and still provide excellent educational reading. Essentially they were medical problems, the talking was done by less than a dozen people, the other 100 or so forming the audience merely listened to the unfolding story and the erudition of the speakers. It never really caught on in Surgery where everyone wanted to join in the discussion and there were few listeners. The C.P.C. demanded a great deal of preparation – any deficiencies soon became evident – and much co-operation between major and busy departments. Even so, a well-managed conference with outstanding performances by the principal actors was a memorable occasion on a Wednesday morning.

At most undergraduate medical schools in London the post-mortem was an obligatory part of training: it was the moment of truth for the clinician who had pontificated about that patient's diagnosis and treatment, and so these occasions were well attended by students who came not always for enlightenment.

POST-MORTEMS

At Hammersmith, post-mortem demonstrations were held at lunch-time and often daily. The most junior doctor attending the patient would provide a brief resumé of the clinical findings and management. The pathologist would demonstrate his macroscopic discoveries, the microscopy when relevant, and a general discussion would ensue.

The whole performance was confined to a group around the corpse: those at the back neither heard nor saw and moved away. When, however, the demonstrations could be held in a lecture theatre it was a different matter: although only selected organs were produced they could be projected by an epidiascope on to a screen for all to see, so that the demonstrator could be questioned and the audience begin to understand. Wolfson II lecture theatre became a focal meeting point for all departments.

Professor Harrison, who had joined the School as an Assistant in Morbid Anatomy in 1935, made these lunch-time meetings his speciality: with a certain ferocity and unwillingness to suffer fools gladly, he had a sense of schoolboy fun and never lost that youthful enthusiasm which he so ably transmitted. Such is the essence of good teaching, and he was an admirable teacher.[75] These demonstrations (or, more correctly, conferences, because all could now join in) were often the occasions for settling old personal scores by asking seemingly innocuous questions, but the occasions were essentially informal: sudden humour or anger could delight and surprise. There were occasions of oratory too. As Nye Bevan once remarked 'the genuine orator, like his peers in other arts, cannot be predicted. He produces his results unexpectedly – quite often as much to himself as to his audience. This quality of spontaneity and immediacy is the very kernel of effective speech.'

As a method of training juniors the post-mortem demonstration was excellent. To have to stand and defend one's opinion and judgement is always salutary: when the opinion is that of one's superior, life can be tough. In the late seventies the number of post-mortems declined, as happened throughout London, and so this method of teaching fell in abeyance.

By then, a different form of teaching, aimed at a national and European audience, had taken over: the 5-day seminar on specific, defined, and often limited subjects usually described as 'recent advances'. The histology to be demonstrated had been transferred to colour transparencies, shown as slides on a large screen, of areas specially selected and stained according to the occasion. Much credit for the correct interpretation of the histology of a specimen examined under a microscope must be accorded to the accuracy and detail of the clinical diagnosis, but even so the quality of the reports from the Department of Pathology at the Hammersmith was exceptionally high and almost certainly because there was an overview system and details were chewed over before utterance. There was also a large referral system, both ways: Hammersmith sent specimens of doubt to those who knew – all over the world, but often to the National Institutes of Health at Bethesda, U.S.A., because that centre had taken the time, trouble and money to build up a reference collection, and many School staff had worked there – because Hammersmith knew they knew and there was equal reciprocity. Few people realized that one pathologist alone was in the habit of examining and reporting on 60 sets of slides a month from outside sources, a considerable load to carry in addition to his normal duties, but invaluable as a store of prestige, goodwill and generosity: the job, like so many others at the Hammersmith, was of course unpaid. The Foundation Professors were astute men, but they were not clairvoyants. Teaching at the School before the war, in general, had followed the principles of undergraduate disciplines: keep the students busy from 10 to 4.30 with 1 hour for lunch, by didactic lectures, collaborative internal meetings, ward rounds, out-patient clinics, and guest lectures by visiting Chiefs to present 'accepted practices' (the way I do things, not why). The short courses changed all that.

In the years 1936 to 1953 the number of U.K. students varied from 225 to 775 annually, and these figures clearly related to 'War Courses'. The seeds of war in Europe were sown the year the School opened: in January the Saar was occupied by Germany and in October Italy invaded Abyssinia. The re-militarization of the Rhineland the next year, and the civil war in Spain in July, put the seal on future conflict. In the same period, 1936–1953, an average of 200 students came from the Commonwealth and a further 100 from other countries abroad. In the past 30 years there has been a noticeable change: fewer doctors have come from Australia, Canada, and New Zealand, but twice the number from foreign countries. The origin of Hammersmith students was as shown in Table 1.

Table 1 Origin of Hammersmith students

Year	*U.K.*	*Commonwealth*	*Foreign countries*	*Total*
1940	283	151	62	496
1953	146	224	110	480
1963	194	192	214	600

Since 1973 there has been a different method of accounting and the popularity of 'short courses' dealing with recent advances in a particular subject became evident (see Table 2).

Table 2 Popularity of short courses

Year	*Total postgraduates*	*Short courses*
1973	1190	691 (59%)
1983	1957	1223 (63%)

Indeed in 1983 the 1223 doctors attended 21 short courses on specialist subjects, of average duration 6 days and average attendance of 59 per course: of these about half came from European countries.

THE HAMMERSMITH TEACHING

How then does teaching at the Hammersmith differ from teaching elsewhere? What makes it 'postgraduate', apart from the fact that the attenders are doctors and not medical students? Finally, in what way has postgraduate teaching evolved in the past 50 years? Sir John McMichael in 1966 made five points[76] about the Hammersmith teaching.

First, 'we teach by example. We can do this by giving an exemplary service and exhibiting this effort to all students who wish to attend, week by week.' this meant emphasizing the quality of the history-taking and clinical examination as well as the precision of the observations. He dismissed the idea that a kind doctor can replace a competent doctor: both are required, but kindness comes second ('even this judgement makes a basic assumption that kindness and cleverness could be mutually exclusive. Nothing could be further from the truth'). Hence medicine must recruit the best available brains in the country (and in most years it does) because these bright cohorts change the whole practice of medicine in the future and make use of all the knowledge we already have.

Second, 'if we teach them the medicine of yesterday this will certainly be of no use to them in a decade or two'. Hammersmith emphasized that problems unravelled by bedside study must be studied in the laboratory so that the understanding of those problems became part of their solution, naturally and axiomatically. It was the accent on medical research that distinguished the School's teaching from that of others.

Third, 'we distil out of our analytical experience, in the wards, postmortem room and laboratory, practical judgements on the best management of the patients and it is this experience that we try to present to all our trainees'. He stated that progressive medicine costs less in money and health than static or second-rate medicine – a view which is still contested and debated today.

Fourth, wisdom. Some people believe it can be acquired by some magical process separate from the way medicine makes use of scientific method. 'Wisdom, however, in my opinion is not attainable without wide-ranging knowledge and we try to make this clear in our teaching which expounds for our students a mode of observation, thought and deduction.'

Fifth, 'the School does not instruct for any examination drill but rather attempts to instill reasoning power. There are no ex cathedra pronouncements. Statements by anybody, senior or junior, are liable to questioning and there is no pretence at omniscience. We study medicine together. . . .' There should be no drudgery in learning, we learn from one another, but there should be a sense of scholarship.

Logical deductions from observations of maximum precision was the recurring theme of the education the School gave: there had never been any distinction between training and education from earliest times and so the advent of the Todd Report in 1968 surprised many. Todd recommended continuing education for all doctors, which the Hammersmith had long accepted as natural. Only paragraphs 453(9) refer directly to Hammersmith: 'We do not in general favour the separation of postgraduate from undergraduate teaching but in the case of the Royal Postgraduate Medical School this seems for the present to be inevitable' – views contrary to those expressed by the Athlone Committee of 1921, the Chamberlain Committee of 1930, the Foundation Professors in 1936, and most of the staff in post in 1968.

Admittedly the terms of reference for the Royal Commission on Medical Education 1965–1968 were to examine undergraduate education, but this included some postgraduate education and training. The pattern recommended after qualification was: an intern year of pre-registration in general medicine and surgery of 6 months each (which was already enforced by the Medical Act of 1950), and general professional training for 3 years; further professional training for a few years which was essentially specialist training; continuing education for all doctors in career posts to keep them abreast of developments. Interestingly, about 2000 final-year students were asked for their views on medical teaching in 1966 by the Commission (Appendix 19 reports the results). Of the 12 possible choices of 'methods of teaching' three – research, lectures, and clinico-pathological conferences, all recognized favourites at Hammersmith – were recorded as the least valuable. Indeed, personal research – the linch-pin of Hammersmith's philosophy of teaching – was the least favoured method!

Sir George Pickering[77], Professor of Medicine at the University of Oxford, later commented in his usual forthright way. 'The idea that education should continue throughout life seems oddly enough, to be novel. It certainly does not gain acceptance in the University of Oxford.' He pointed out that although the Final Honours course of only 3 years set out to train a man to be fit for independent research in his subject, about half the men on the arts side come to Oxford with no knowledge of science and left with none. 'The University seems to specialise in turning out ignorant men.'

EDUCATION AND TRAINING

A distinction has to be made between education and training; training is vocational and concerned to bring a man to a desired standard of efficiency by instruction and practice; education is a process by which an individual is encouraged to develop the powers of his mind, to discover, to assimilate, to criticize and to synthesize, and the process is stimulated by teachers and contemporaries who themselves display these qualities. Training and education were considered complementary to each other and had proceeded together at the Hammersmith: it was really the organizational structure of the National Health Service which tended to separate them. Training is the perfection of skills, of patterns of reaction to situations that frequently recur, and implies that certain tasks shall be done often and under critical surveillance – learning by doing is the central theme – hence the succession of posts from house officer to senior registrar, allowing progressive responsibility with increasing seniority. But as Pickering and MacLachlan noted[78]: 'The consultant, by contrast, has no surveillance other than his conscience and the judgement of his peers.'

In the N.H.S. there are competing claims of training and service. The Postgraduate School originally set out to train doctors for general practice but after the war concentrated on training specialists – the 1948 N.H.S. Act was essentially a hospital-based Act – and only in 1983 was the Regional Adviser in General Practice located at the School. Indeed, in 1961, postgraduate education in the U.K. was almost entirely confined to that for specialists and foreigners: it was provided by the teaching hospitals and the British Postgraduate Medical Federation of which the Hammersmith was the largest unit and the only general hospital. Yet, educational and service needs in the N.H.S. are inextricably mixed, although many have tried to separate them and failed.

In the U.S.A. and for most of Europe, the qualifying examination is M.D. It means 'safe to practise'. Specialist training may follow after a period of general experience, usually in hospital, and competence is assessed by Specialty Boards: a certificate is awarded, can be hung on the office wall, and the recipient is free to earn his living as a specialist in a particular subject.

In Britain the qualification for 'safe to practise' is M.B., B.S. (or similar), the titles M.D. and M.S. being reserved for higher degrees awarded by a university. In order to qualify for specialist training the doctor must sit a further examination at a minimum time after qualification, the diploma being awarded not by a university but by one of the Colleges: F.R.C.S., M.R.C.P., M.R.C.O.G., M.R.C.G.P., M.R.C.Path., M.R.C.Psych., and so on. The specialist training status is Senior Registrar at an 'approved' post for 3 years, at the end of which the individual receives a certificate of accreditation and becomes eligible to apply for a vacant post as consultant in the N.H.S. Posts in hospitals are approved by the College's Specialty Committee on the number of beds allocated to that specialty, the number of consultants working there, the volume and variety of patients being seen and treated. The duration of training as a Senior Registrar may be reduced by tenure as Registrar in that specialty and by a period devoted to research: usually the combined concession must not exceed 18 months. Because of these rather rigid limitations by which a doctor can become a hospital consultant or general practitioner in the N.H.S. there is little inducement for any trainee to increase his breadth or depth of knowledge from the kind of research and clinical work that Hammersmith offered. Not only have career prospects deteriorated in the past 10 years, but the age at appointment has steadily increased: in popular specialties the average age to a consultant post, admittedly a job for life, is now

38 in surgery and medicine. Moreover, to be certain of a place in the queue for training, doctors at Senior House Officer grade compete to join specialist units. This whole method of self-selection is contrary to the Hammersmith view of postgraduate medical education.

In the words of McMichael: 'Interest in medicine arises from the effort we make to understand the phenomena before our eyes. Effort is rewarded by intellectual enjoyment. Hard work generates interest and hard work in medicine is always, to my mind rewarded.' When that was written in 1966, the School had able and idealistic young men who felt that the challenge of academic work was more attractive than the better financial rewards available outside the Medical School. In 1984 there is evidence of a change of attitude and a demand for the 'market price' of the expertise that the Hammersmith can offer.

Ten years after the Royal Commission on Medical Education very few of its recommendations had been implemented because the University budget for medicine had grown from 30% in 1969 to 35% in 1979 of the total resources, was continuing to rise, and so a working party was set up under the chairmanship of Lord Flowers.[79] The report, 'London Medical Education – a New Framework', published in February 1980, created controversy. Flowers recommended that the present 34 separate establishments be grouped into six Schools of Medicine and Dentistry in London. The 'twinning' of medical schools recommended by Lord Todd had not been achieved: the idea had been to reduce the 12 medical schools to six, but 10 years later the new St George's and the new Charing Cross Hospitals and Medical Schools were firmly established as single entities on new sites and with different responsibilities to the National Health Service which had supplied the money to rebuild the hospitals.

Both Reports, Todd in 1968 and Flowers in 1980, were concerned mainly with undergraduate education, but both made comments on postgraduate education as though the two went together quite naturally; both reports were concerned with London where the number of final-year medical students (568 in 1966) was more than the sum of those in the rest of England, Wales and Scotland. Both Todd and Flowers agreed that each of the 12 specialties of the Postgraduate Federation (where there were 4625 hospital beds in 1967) should be linked to, or better incorporated into, a general hospital on the grounds that 'isolation' was bad for 'standards', without defining these terms. Todd did not like the idea of the Hammersmith, the only general hospital for postgraduate studies in the U.K. then and today, being separated from undergraduate teaching, but accepted that it seemed inevitable.

The Flowers report conceded that the Hammersmith was unique in the way it was organized, recognized that the School and Hospital 'have a national and international reputation and provide a wide range of medical specialties for patients from the immediate locality and for referrals from other parts of the country and abroad', accepted that half the students came from abroad to spend varying periods at the School, but then recommended that 'Just as basic medical education should be integrated with clinical instruction, so postgraduate medical education should be an on-going process following the undergraduate years.' At that time there was no evidence that mixing basic education with clinical work, in a form of vertical integration, had produced better doctors than those who had learned their basic subjects (of anatomy, physiology, pharmacology) before starting clinical work; nor is there sufficient evidence in 1984. Flowers did not appear to understand that postgraduate education at the Hammersmith differed from postgraduate education elsewhere, in the integration of teaching, research and clinical care by full-time University doctors, and was likely to continue to be different because in the past 50 years no other School or Hospital had even attempted the same sort of organization. The Report continued 'It will be to the advantage of both for postgraduate and undergraduate education to come together', but produced no evidence to support this claim. It proposed that the Hammersmith should formally link with St Mary's Medical School, and the Institute of Dental Surgery (the Eastman Dental Hospital). The Royal Postgraduate Medical School rejected the link and in May 1980 asked the University for adequate finance to remain independent, but to continue the links with the Institute of Child Health, the Institute of Obstetrics, and to explore a research link with Imperial College (in fact a link had been established a decade earlier but had never flourished).

The arguments were by no means over. In October of the same year the Report of the Joint Planning Committee of the Court and the Senate of the University, 'Medical Education in London', recorded that the R.P.M.S. was 'the best known international centre of general medical research within the University. It has received massive support for its research activities and attracts from the MRC more than double the sum (£2.66 M in 1978–79) for research, including direct support units, than any other School in the University. The R.P.M.S. holds, therefore, a special place of prestige in the University and, if it were to be unable to operate, the loss to medical research in this country would be deplorable.' Note the accent on research, whereas Flowers had emphasized teaching, but also in contrast the concluding sentence: 'No union with St. Mary's HMS or any other Medical School would improve its financial situation.' The report noted that the R.P.M.S. was undeniably expensive for the University because the vast majority of consultant staff at Hammersmith Hospital – and hospitals were always considered as N.H.S. liabilities even if medical schools depended for their survival on patients in these hospitals – are academics paid from University funds. 'Its funding must be raised with the Government and a detailed case made out for a special recurrent grant . . . and that the 1951 Agreement for consultant staffing be re-examined with the Department (the DHSS).' It seemed that at last a committee had recognized that teaching, research and education in medicine were a joint responsibility of the University and the

National Health Service, not only in London but in the country as a whole, and that the decisions of one affected the other.

The Joint Planning Committee recommended that their report be adopted as the policy of the University on the future of medical education in the University and that the proposals be implemented. In November 1981 Final Proposals were published. St Mary's Hospital Medical School would continue as a strong independent unit with academic links to the Royal Postgraduate Medical School. In the reorganization of the National Health Service of 1982, Hammersmith Hospital became a Special Health Authority directly accountable to the Minister of Health, but for other administrative problems it was included in the North West Thames Regional Health Authority. Although considerable progress had been made in recognizing Hammersmith's contribution to medical education it was unlikely that it had ever been really understood by those not intimately involved. Education for doctors will be debated for a long time to come. Tout expliquer, c'est tout détruire: perhaps Madame de Stael had spoken the truth.

12

Research

In medicine, in its widest sense, there has always been a reasonably clear distinction between scholarship and research. Scholarship meant keeping abreast of the current state of one's own subject and those which are closest to it; this may include writing books and papers which expound and systematize what is known. The School did just that during its formative years from 1935 until after the war. Research, on the other hand, meant advancing what is known and uncovering the unknown: this process began in the School during the war years but did not blossom until much later. It is axiomatic that scholarship is part of the duty of every teacher in medicine, and that postgraduate institutions must make adequate provision for scholarship, including provision of libraries and for travel. Research in many branches of medicine can be expensive, and in general is not viewed by others as an essential element of teaching in the same way that those at the Hammersmith insisted it was. For this reason there was real fear that research would suffer irreparably when financial stringency affected the School in the late seventies: that it did not is testimony to the strength of the Hammersmith tradition.

However, in research, the largest component by far is the thinking time of the staff, which is difficult to quantify, but can be safeguarded by making staff posts full-time. That is what the Hammersmith and the University wanted, but the time came when the University could no longer pay for all the staff that Hammersmith demanded. As a result, from 1970 onwards, an increasing number of researchers were paid by the N.H.S. for their service commitment to patients and by the School for their teaching and research.

As money got tighter, research suffered: time to think went first. All researchers at Hammersmith were amateurs in the sense that each had a lasting passion for asking questions and finding answers. Research at the Hammersmith was done not as a duty or a wage-earning job but as an exciting piece of detective work by a practising clinician which led to publication, recognition, advancement of knowledge and of career too. Everyone took part, and all started equal. It is commonly stated that research is largely a matter of having an original idea, presenting it as a question, and then searching for the answer. Hammersmith understood how difficult it was to create a new idea and the enormous odds against such an event. It knew that the right environment helped and the Foundation Professors tried to provide that; they also grabbed anyone with a new concept and were tolerant if he did not ask the right question immediately. The four Professors brought their own research interests with them: Fraser (thyroid disease, myasthenia gravis), Turner (oesophageal cancer and bladder abnormalities), Young (nutrition in pregnancy, foetal mortality), Kettle (silicosis, lung disease). Some lines were pursued by their successors, others abandoned. But there was nothing peculiarly Hammersmith about the research except that good doctors were, rather surprisingly, doing it and doing it well while running a general hospital.

What the Foundation Professors brought to the School was not outstanding research ability, but leadership. Indeed the quantity and quality of research at the Hammersmith from 1935 to 1941 was small. They believed that success in research would be achieved by leadership and not by a committee or by governmental directives (and hence their suspiciousness of the National Health Service in 1948). They believed that a man of courage and vision and experience was required at the head of the enterprise to tell the researchers what to study, where to look and for what purpose. Participation, democracy, group dynamics, joint consultation and so on (which the N.H.S. promised, and which was in keeping with Parliamentary practices) were all very well, but someone had to point the way and that same person had to ensure that everyone concerned got there. Organizational effectiveness depended on the quality of leadership: there was no substitute.

THE 1944 RECOMMENDATIONS

The Goodenough Report[80] recorded that 'Medical Schools, teaching hospitals and postgraduate institutes have three important functions in relation to medical research: to discover and train future research workers; to encourage and facilitate original investigations by members of their teaching staffs; and to house special research units and workers'. Hammersmith did all three. On the organization of research workers, Goodenough stated:

- Innumerable problems of health and disease are awaiting solution.
- A community that wishes to promote research must first find and train the men who have the ability and the impulse for scientific enquiry. It must

then create the most favourable conditions for their work and give them the tools they need.

- Young research workers should mainly recruit themselves, their careers being closely watched and guided.
- When a worker has proved his research ability and has chosen research as a career, he should be given reasonable security in his career.
- Scientific workers in other than medical fields have a valuable contribution to make to medical research.

'Apart from basic grants (that is public grants for research to medical schools), extra grants will be needed from public and private sources for the support of special investigations by regular members of the staffs of teaching centres and research workers attached to the centres specially for the purpose'. That the Committee's ideas about research should mirror the thinking at Hammersmith at that time was surprising, but not all the recommendations of Goodenough were achieved quickly and some were too altruistic.

In 1941 Bywaters, a Beit Research Fellow and Part-time Assistant in the Department of Medicine (and allowed to examine patients at other hospitals) made the simple observation that people buried under rubble during air raids often died from kidney failure without any obvious reason. It was in the School that the clinical picture of renal failure following upon an injury was clearly appreciated, and the full clinical and biochemical picture of the 'crush syndrome' was worked out; it was published by Bywaters and Beall in the *British Medical Journal* in 1941. A vast mass of work had been undertaken by Bywaters and most of the School staff. More papers followed in 1942–1944 with Professor Dible and Dr Popjak, and Bywaters was directed to take charge of a Medical Research Council Trauma Unit in Newcastle in January 1944, but returned to London early in 1945. His Beit Trust Grant had been extended to a fourth year in 1942 to allow him to continue the work experimentally: he found, in rabbits, that the crushing of muscle alone did not produce renal failure but that the subsequent injection of myohaemoglobin did.

Bywaters[81] (whose main interest was in rheumatism and joint disease) did more than describe a fatal and puzzling condition that had been highlighted by air-raid casualties; his work united all the Foundation Departments in the first communal research project, and established a process whereby future Hammersmith research would be conducted: the problem is identified – lead tests are performed – the condition is reproduced in animals to allow detailed study – possible methods of treatment are attempted in animals – treatment is then transferred to patients – difficulties or unexpected results are returned to the laboratory for elucidation – the solution is referred back to the bedside – and so on. This technique of a shuttle between laboratory-experiment and patient-illness was to be used subsequently and successfully for the Melrose heart–lung machine, a polypropylene artificial mitral heart valve, for artificial finger joints, and many other developments.

EARLY CLINICAL RESEARCH

The move away from case reports of rare diseases towards general medical physiology marked the beginning of a new concept in clinical research for the twentieth century. Indeed, once a problem was known and understood it was often a straightforward matter to develop countermeasures. In 1947 Dr W. J. Kolff from Holland, donated one of his early kidney dialysis machines – for years it remained in the School workshop, a monument and museum piece – and an assistant to manage it, Dr A. M. Joekes, who stayed for 2 years. By 1948 patients with barbiturate poisoning, a common and highly effective method of suicide at the time, were being treated successfully on the 'artificial kidney' but interest was moving inevitably towards the study of renal blood flow.

The Department of Medicine report for 1944 specifically mentions two areas of research which were being developed as special interests ('in spite of flying bombs and rockets'): the circulation and liver disease. McMichael, who had been Reader in Medicine since 1939, developed an auricular catheter technique (with his First Assistant, Dr E. P. Sharpey-Schafer[82]) to study cardiac output in man in shock, blood loss and heart disease. Great advances in knowledge were made: they were later joined by Dr Sheila Howarth and a visiting research worker (Dr O. G. Edholm, who a year later became Professor) who measured intracardiac pressures, studied heart failure in Paget's Disease, anaemia and even arteriovenous aneurysms. The team was later joined by many well-known names in cardiology, and the tradition of interest has continued to the present time.

In 1942 Dr Sheila Sherlock,[83] who had joined the staff as a research assistant under the aegis of the Medical Research Council's Jaundice Committee to study liver disease, developed a needle biopsy technique so that the results of liver function tests and histology could be examined at the same time: the first result was that there appeared to be two types of liver lesion in heart failure: one anoxic in origin, the other from high venous pressure. McMichael in the annual report for 1944 wrote: 'Her courage in the development of the technique of liver biopsy has been rewarded by a complete absence of any complications in over 100 aspirations. This work is throwing new light on liver function tests and will make a formidable contribution to medical knowledge'. It did. Sherlock was appointed Beit Research Fellow in 1944. Subsequently, her pioneer work and that of McMichael were severely criticized as unethical.[84] By 1947 there were six areas of research in the Department which covered cardiovascular, respiratory, renal, endocrine, rheumatism, liver and metabolic diseases. These represented the areas of research which interested the various people working in the Department, who in effect were clinicians for the Hospital and researchers for the school: their reputations for either activity rested on both.

Almost by contrast, the Department of Surgery contracted. Three First Assistants (Ruscoe Clark, Donald Douglas, and R. T. Payne), one Assistant (Ivor Griffiths) and the Reader in Surgery (A. K. Henry) were away on war service and research had virtually to be abandoned. There was a heavy clinical load on those remaining at the Hammersmith: in 1940 it was usual to receive 20–30 patients after an air raid, but in 1944 during the time of the flying bombs and rockets there could be as many as 85 casualties treated in one night. When war ceased, Aird took over the Chair of Surgery from Grey Turner in 1946: Turner had been there for 11 years and was now 69 years old, yet had done his stint of operations as well as running most of the organized teaching. Even by 1947 the surgical staff were mainly recent appointees and more concerned with clinical practice than research, but in that year Dempster[85] was appointed Leverhulme Fellow, resident at the Buxton Browne Farm of the Royal College of Surgeons, to begin research on organ transplantation: the investigation of renal function by Ralph Shackman[86] (who had spent a year with Blalock in the U.S.A.), and of fluid mechanics for organ perfusion (soon to develop into a heart–lung machine) by Denis Melrose[87] followed in 1949.

In Pathology, a Department which from the beginning was based on the four separate disciplines of morbid anatomy, biochemistry, bacteriology and haematology, a great deal of collaborative research occurred within the School: Beall, Dible, King, Macfarlane, Janet Vaughan, Stamp, Belt, Haslewood, Harrison were all publishing papers on important subjects in 1939. The Department was also the only section of the School to run an integrated diploma course (for the D.C.P.), and during the war taught pathology to undergraduates from St Mary's and the West London Hospital. Traumatic anuria was the one subject which united all subdivisions of that department from 1942 to 1944: by 1948 each unit had in effect become autonomous, and the amount of routine work for hospital patients had increased.

The Department of Obstetrics and Gynaecology had 124 beds, for about 2000 confinements a year, and was responsible for paediatrics. Thirty-seven beds were set aside for women suffering from the complications of pregnancy (such as toxaemia, haemorrhage, heart disease, and disproportion): in 1939, 500 such cases were admitted. Dr Alan Moncrieff,[88] the Consultant in Paediatrics, visited once a week: it was not until 1945 that he became Professor of Child Health in the University, with 'duties at the British Postgraduate Medical School and The Hospital for Sick Children, Great Ormond Street' – a link which remains today – and the appointments of a Registrar and First Assistant for care of the newborn in the Obstetric Unit were made. Research in O & G tended to be clinical: the use of penicillin in labour and abortion, the effect of analgesic agents on mother and child, caudal anaesthesia for the relief of pelvic pain.

By 1948, a Premature Baby Unit was opened with 20 cots (and six beds for mothers). Mollison had carried out successfully 16 replacement transfusions on newborn infants for erythroblastosis foetalis, and the Department was incorporated into a combined teaching school with Queen Charlotte's Hospital and the Chelsea Hospital for Women to form a recognized and independent institute of the British Postgraduate Medical Federation (The Institute of Obstetrics and Gynaecology). This Institute, which had been threatened with abolition in the Todd Report of 1968 and the Flowers Report of 1980, eventually rejoined the Hammersmith on 1 April 1984, the whole to be known as the 'Hammersmith and Queen Charlotte's Special Health Authority' – an N.H.S. reorganization rather than a University one.

Paediatrics started as a sub-unit of the Department of Obstetrics (the association of mother and child was logical) but when the Postgraduate Medical Federation was formed in 1947 each went separate ways: the former joined with Chelsea and Queen Charlotte's Hospitals to form the Institute of Obstetrics and Gynaecology based at Dove Street, the latter with the Institute of Child Health based at Great Ormond Street. In practice, every baby born at Hammersmith Hospital was inspected by a paediatrician before discharge home, but administratively and organizationally they had separated.

The School could not ignore the unit of paediatrics on site, particularly when collaborative research with other academic departments on the problems of the newborn drew world attention, but it was not until 1963 that paediatrics was given the status of a Department. Tizard, who had been head of the unit since 1954, was made Professor in 1964 with Dawkins (who died at the early age of 34) and Davies as Lecturers: the latter became Reader the following year and in 1967 moved to Manchester as Professor of Paediatrics. Five years later Tizard[89] became the first Professor of Paediatrics at the University of Oxford, to be succeeded by Dubowitz whose main interest was in muscle disorders. Charles Newman, who had acted as Consultant Paediatrician to Hammersmith Hospital as well as Dean of the School since 1940, retired when the Department was recognized.

RESEARCH FUNDING

The National Health Service had supplied monies for research since its inception, but in diverse ways and in small amounts. The funds most relevant to the Hammersmith were those of the Locally Organized Research Scheme (L.O.R.S.) which succeeded the Locally Organized Clinical Research Scheme (of the early fifties) in May 1975 when the department of Health established a central fund and issued a code of practice. In 1978 the administration of the scheme was devolved to the 14 Regional Health Authorities and Board of Governors of the various teaching and special hospitals: many of the latter accepted to join the Regional schemes. The central monies of £2.4 million were distributed in 1978 to the Regions and were included in their total revenue allocations: greatly to their credit most Regions, at a time of severe financial constraints and general unrest with pay and conditions in the N.H.S. in the late seventies and early eighties, decided to continue to allocate the same proportion of the money to research as was allotted in 1978 and to retain the values of the total.

When Hammersmith Hospital became a Special Health Authority in 1982, over £90,000 was ceded from the North-West Thames Regional Health Authority, to which the Hospital had formally belonged, as a reasonable amount to hand over. The Trustees of the Special Health Authority Fund chipped in with monies from endowments to make the total to around £120,000, equivalent to 0.05% of the total Hospital budget and thus in line with the proportions supplied by Regions. The total monies spent by all 14 Regional Health Authorities in England in 1982/1983 were £4.16 million, rather less than the Hammersmith Staff raised by personal effort. However, the Locally Organized Research Scheme budget monies do allow newcomers to research, particularly junior hospital staff, to get projects started before applying to the major grant-giving bodies such as the Medical Research Council, Wellcome Trust, Nuffield Foundation and the many other generous donors recorded in the annual reports of the Royal Postgraduate Medical School. The aim of the L.O.R.S. was to 'foster the research spirit in the health profession which is conducive to a high standard of practice, and to facilitate the discovery and encouragement of local talent'. No-one could quarrel with these sentiments, but Hammersmith wanted money in much greater amounts.

One of the features of the annual reports of the School is the list of 'Grants and benefactions during the year'. Almost all are for research and are often referred to as 'soft monies', an error of terminology if ever there was because these monies represent grants for specific research projects awarded to a particular member of staff who applied, in open competition countrywide, and with scientific merit as the sole criterion of success. It is a form of competition for realistic ideas, beneficial to donor and recipient, which has done much to advance the quality of medical practice: it is also hard work and time-consuming, but provides a certain satisfaction when successful.

The Annual Report of the Postgraduate Medical School of London for the year 1952–1953 (almost as an afterthought and printed on the inside back cover) for the first time listed the 18 grants received from 10 separate bodies (it was a beginning even though the Medical Research Council made 9 of the 18 grants).

The amount of money raised by staff members has increased considerably over the years, as Table 3 demonstrates.

The School's basic financial support has derived always from the University Grants Committee, a Government agency which distributes Exchequer funds to all universities. Most of the research work is funded from competitive grants awarded by many bodies and these are by nature short-term grants – of 3–5 years or less – which implied that there had to be a continuous input of new ideas by staff in order to preserve the income (which may be no bad thing,

Table 3

	1939	*1953*	*1983*
Total School income	£56,730	£247,317	£11.7 million
University of London Grant	83%	69%	39%
National Health Service	3% (LCC)	16%	15%
Tuition fees from students	13%	3%	8%
Interest on endowments	1%	2%	1%
Grants for specific research projects	—	10%	37%

but allowed little scope for long-term planning). The N.H.S. monies paid for work done in the School's laboratories (mainly in pathology, biochemistry, bacteriology and haematology) thus saving the Hospital the need to provide these essential services. Whichever way one looks at it, the effort by staff to obtain grants and benefactions almost equal to those from the University was a significant contribution to the School's economy and a remarkable achievement. In the 10 years 1973–1983 the grant income climbed from £774,000 to £4.9 million. In these 10 years accounting systems had changed three times and so the figure for 1982–1983 does not tally with the published total of £3.1 million for itemized grants in the annual report of that year. Nevertheless, the figures are impressive but they are figures in isolation: they ignore inflation, other income, which staff raised most money, and which grant-giving bodies headed the list.

GRANTS VALUE AND AGENCIES

The conventional cost of living index has rarely applied to medicine and never to the Hammersmith. Indeed the cost of living index is fine for preserving the status quo (if there is such a thing) but no good at all when it comes to scientific equipment and advances in medicine. According to Whitaker the purchasing power of £1 in 1973 is comparable to £3.43 in 1982 and this can be used as an index of the cost of living. Alternatively, according to the Department of Employment calculations, from 1970 to 1980, wages rose by 400%, Consultant salaries by 300% and the Retail Price Index by 350% (*Whitaker's Almanac* for 1984 quotes 320%).

Using these criteria in 1983 the income from grant applications by staff was ahead of inflation by a factor of two, while the University grant money was exactly level and so had not increased in real terms. The services supplied to the Hospital (the bill for services tended to be nominal, but was agreed by bargaining) in 1973 was £390,000 and in 1982 £1.730 million, an increase greater than the rate of inflation. In addition the School received income from private patient fees, investments and miscellaneous sources which rose from £85,000 to £297,000 during this period and roughly in line with inflation. It is therefore clear that the main source of income for the School came from the University of London (monies which paid the salaries of academic staff) and from individual grants (which paid for research, including staff and equipment). It was equally clear that in 1983, staff earned 62% of the total School income.

As already recorded, the Medical Research Council (M.R.C.) contributed heavily to research grants in the early post-war period of the School. For the past 10 years (1973–1974 to 1982–1983) the M.R.C. had consistently supplied 30% of the total school research monies. The M.R.C. is the main government agency for the support of biomedical research, and has over 50 research units mostly located in university departments, medical schools and hospitals in Britain. It runs two major research institutes, at Mill Hill and the Clinical Research Centre at Northwick Park, a mere 12 miles from the Hammersmith. The fact that monies from the M.R.C. were granted to staff at the Hammersmith must to some extent be seen as an endorsement of the excellence of the ideas presented for research, and the fact that grants continued as evidence that the research was well done. In 10 years the M.R.C. supplied over £5.5 million.

One other agency had consistently supported research most generously (and in other ways, some of which have already been noted, such as the library, laboratory buildings, travel grants): the Wellcome Trust. In the 10 years 1973–1974 to 1982–1983 this Trust had made grants of nearly £3 million on an average of 30 applications annually, representing a consistent 15% of the School's income for research. Others are beginning to catch up: for instance the British Heart Foundation which endowed a Chair of Cardiology in 1976 (the first Sir John McMichael Chair of Cardiovascular Medicine: Shillingford the incumbent until 1979, Maseri followed) and a further Chair of Cardiac Surgery in 1983 (Taylor was appointed in August), also contributed £171,293 in 12 individual research grants.[90]

Undoubtedly the largest share of grant money for research comes under the heading of 'others', an impressive total of over £18 million in the 10 years to 1982–1983, in response to an average of about 100 applications a year. The donors have varied from well-known pharmaceutical companies to quite minor charities. The most consistent has been Smith's Charity, which first gave money in 1952 and 30 years later continues, sometimes for specific areas of interest ('for arthritis research') but commonly as a donation to general funds. Without all these 'grants and benefactions' the School would have been a fairly sterile place. The vast majority of grants, and the largest individual sums requested, have come from about half-a-dozen individuals in the various disciplines of medicine, pharmacology, immunology, and cell biology. The outward signs of active research are money and publications; they go together, and it requires a certain amount of flair to keep the two in tune.

HAMMERSMITH AIMS OF RESEARCH

The Hammersmith encouraged everyone to do research, preferably their own project, but they could join in what was already under way, and writing a thesis was accepted as a reasonable aim. Hammersmith provided a good environment for research if only because it was the normal thing to do and everyone else was thus engaged. Money was not provided: the financing of research was left to the individual. It was possible to seek advice on how to apply successfully for funds – there was always a guru on site – and one was taught research techniques. The object of research at the Hammersmith is often ill-understood. The School has no Nobel Prize winners (except the current President, Sir Peter Medawar, who was awarded the Nobel Prize for Medicine in 1960) and very few Fellows of the Royal Society (F.R.S.), both of which are commonly taken as measurement of the 'quality' and 'importance' of research being done. In 1935 there were four professors and two F.R.S; 50 years later there are 28 professors and three F.R.S. Research was a discipline used to develop courage, dedication and leadership in medicine and in that respect has been highly successful. In the U.K. there is not a single specialty nor a teaching hospital where Hammersmith graduates have not introduced this 'culture' to the advantage of both.

Research at the Hammersmith revolved around patients, directly by attending physicians and surgeons, indirectly by service departments (such as pathology or radiology: there were never more than a handful of full-time staff researchers) and had three aims.

First, to unravel clinical problems: the diagnosis, treatment, natural history, the evaluation and assessment of all aspects of general management of the patient and his disease. To be able to carry out this duty Hammersmith believed that good research was necessary and fundamental to the process. There were many 'firsts' (and seconds and thirds) in advancing clinical practice but the main thrust was in the understanding and development of new conceptual ideas: the gut as an endocrine organ, or the electric heart would have been silly titles for conferences 20 years earlier, but in 1983 were thought natural.

Second, as a basic training so that what was discovered by understanding one disease could be used in the investigation of another: the point was to develop imagination and acquire the habit of intellectual detachment.

Third, as the basis for teaching 'true medicine' and as a method of monitoring what was taught at Hammersmith and elsewhere, particularly the latter.

Research has always depended on men and women with ideas and scientific ability, on time, money and facilities, on the close collaboration between individual departments and institutions. Hammersmith had been fortunate in attracting the right people and for the past 20 years all research units have collaborated with units outside the School, very often in different countries. By 1983 Hammersmith research had inevitably become multinational and multidisciplined: a view of 'the wider world' that was shared as more visitors joined for a sabbatical year from the U.S.A., Canada, Australia and Europe.

The rich tapestry of research in the eighties is difficult to describe and condense into a few pages. Open at random a medical textbook of any specialty and the subject on that page is likely to be, or to have been, the focus of attention of Hammersmith researchers. In the sixties it was common to find one subject, say bone density, being studied by six different people (radiologist, endocrinologist, plastic surgeon, orthopaedic surgeon, rheumatologist, biochemist) by different techniques and with different aims. In 1980, single techniques of research worked out earlier were used by many: the identification of enzymes (histochemistry) and of monoclonal antibodies (immunology) had become commonplace in almost every unit. The change is reflected in staff publications. In 1973, of the 560 published papers 10% represented interdepartmental collaborative work: in 1983, 30% of the 826 publications were of joint research by different departments in the School or elsewhere, a significant change of practice. Hammersmith's research can be summarized as in Table 4.

Table 4 Hammersmith research

Year	*Number of autonomous units doing research*	*Number of separate items of research*	*Number of publications for that year*
1953	10	76	271
1963	31	135	346
1973	52	233	560
1983	41	318	826

Anthony Sampson, author of *The Changing Anatomy of Britain*, wrote of scientists 'who can spend so much time with so little to show for it', also noted that 'Governments which pay for more than half their country's research have repeatedly tried to pin down scientists to national objectives'. He missed one essential point. Creativity depends on one person who starts with a new idea and persists with it. Lord Rothschild's Report of 1971 at the Think Tank was based on big industrial organizations like Shell – about as far removed from the Hammersmith confederate-type of research as it is possible to be – and had little relevance to medicine. Rothschild stated: 'The customer says what he wants: the contractor does it (if he can) and the customer pays.' The real trouble was that the customer usually did not know what he wanted by way of research. What the customer wanted was the opportunity to choose between a couple of alternatives and to be fully informed of the cost and consequences of each. But real life is rarely like that. Sampson wrote that 'scientists have resented every infringement of their freedom, while communication between the two sides (i.e. the politicians and the scientists) remained rudimentary'. Certainly communication has not improved in the past 20 years, partly because no Minister of Health has remained in post long enough for there to be a meaningful and trusting dialogue.[91]

13

Clinical Practice

At most of the 12 voluntary hospitals with medical schools in 1935 London – accommodating about 3000 medical students in training – the consultants who worked and taught there were part-time. The senior surgeon or physician was nominally head of his discipline and jealous of his position. Professors were unusual, even in pathology where the work was also part-time: in the provincial universities full-time pathologists were common. The appointment of four full-time Professors to a hospital in London in 1935 was therefore novel. The three Professors of medicine, surgery and gynaecology were considered to hold 'clinical' posts: each had a Reader, two first Assistants, about four housemen and 150 beds.

The Professor of Pathology was considered to be 'non-clinical' and was paid less than his colleagues. But he did have four Readers – one each in the subjects of morbid anatomy, bacteriology, chemical pathology and haematology, and of course all were full-time appointments – and four to six Assistants. There were no beds and so no housemen: the seniors did the work, wrote the reports and were accountable for their opinions. As a result there was a dearth of experienced pathologists in junior grades, as there is even today. The distinction between 'clinical' and 'non-clinical' was considered irrelevant at the Hammersmith – the back-up by the pathologist allowed the clinician to do his job better – for all were concerned with the welfare of patients. As if to emphasize the unity of ward and laboratory, Fraser and Kettle introduced the regular monthly clinico-pathological conferences to Hammersmith, occasions when the patient's symptoms and signs were matched with the pathological findings, for the instruction of everyone. At the weekly staff rounds, a pathologist was always present.

The Foundation Professors brought physiology to the bedside. They were concerned with pumps and pressures, flows and filters, and if one asked what did Hammersmith do better than any other hospital the answer must be 'diagnosis'. Whole-time clinicians, involved in teaching and research and supported by whole-time pathologists similarly engaged, could not help but became outstanding.[92] Later, the back-up included many specialist clinical subjects to ensure that the Hammersmith continued to excel in diagnosis even though there had been a shift to 'molecular biology at the bed side' (genes, cellular changes, immune systems and antibody diversity, a completely new view of infections, and risk factors).

The main reason for acquiring a postgraduate centre of medical education in London was to train better doctors. Hence the Foundation Professors and Readers were hand-picked for their excellence as practitioners by an appointments committee that included the top doctors in the country. Likewise, the Professors in selecting their own staff had to follow suit. Doctors who are going to teach other doctors must be judged in all that they do by their peers (that is, those of equal ability to be able to judge) in the same way that a commercial organization is judged by its profits and a researcher by his publications. It is not enough to be judged by patient satisfaction, important though that is. From early days medical staff were appointed on three qualities. First the need to be good at their job, well-qualified and knowledgeable. Second, they must be aware of advances and up-to-date in details. Third, they should contribute to advances by setting standards, developing special expertise, and becoming innovators.[93]

Innovation is the life-blood of any organization. There is nothing so stultifying to an institute – that is to the people in it – as a belief that the old ways must be the best ways: an organization which tries to stand still does not survive and the Hammersmith had no intention of standing still. Innovation requires a blend of creativity, clear thinking, and the ability to get things done: it demands that thinkers and doers must work closely together. The Professors, as heads of departments, created the climate in which doctors had scope to develop new ideas and the resources to develop them. In the end, the success of innovative projects invariably depended on two things: the characteristics of the individual Professors and the climate of the organization; at Hammersmith both were good. Clinical practice, like the research at Hammersmith, had never been deciding what should be done and then getting others to do it. An enquiring mind, independent spirit, initiative and innovation were the qualities that the Foundation Professors looked for in appointing staff to the School. There were to be found in research posts rather than in routine clinical posts, and independent operating without specific guidelines was essential in the early days although no-one had attempted to define what was meant by research. Was it to be the acquisition of new knowledge for its own sake? Or only useful knowledge? Or even just facts?

CLINICAL PRACTICE ATTITUDES

Hammersmith interpreted the directive (to develop postgraduate medicine) in two distinct ways: an attitude of mind to the patient and a specific problem related to disease such as treatment. The creative and investigative sides were to be amalgamated, and the incentive for success was to be achievement. Research is coolly intellectual, not warmly emotional as much clinical practice must be, and because they tend to be different, many doctors failed to understand that good clinical practice and good research could be done by the same person. Yet the advantages were obvious: research made the clinician better at his job because he was continually seeking answers to why and why not. The patient, inevitably, benefited from the intellectual analysis of his symptoms, signs and response to treatment. The research clinician was doing two things at the same time: he was treating his patient and exploring the disease. The same three qualities that were needed in teaching and research are also needed in clinical practice: courage, patience, and sensitivity. Hammersmith knew this instinctively and never tried to separate research from clinical practice unless there was some corporate advantage to be gained. McMichael once commented 'the research opportunities that arise from the day-to-day treatment of patients are not always appreciated by others', and again 'the alert clinician is the most lively researcher with feet on the ground for practical issues and head in the clouds for imaginative concepts'.

Yet there was criticism of this attitude to medical practice. As pioneers the staff of the School were exposed to a lot of criticism: over liver biopsies, cardiac catheterization, kidney transplants and a whole host of others. The pioneering days were stressful: two examples will suffice. The School's interest in cardiac catheterization and estimation of pulmonary volume led to the introduction of cardiac surgery on site, but the real advances would come from the ability to operate on a still heart. Aird believed that such was possible, but Melrose had first to develop a by-pass pump at Downe (Darwin's old home in Kent) and solve the problem of sterilizing such a large piece of equipment. Even the Medical Research Council thought the project not possible, and it was the Nuffield Foundation that provided finance for the work to continue. Even when animal experiments had shown that satisfactory perfusion of the whole body was possible the problems remained of selecting the first patient. In medicine it is usual to select a patient who is almost moribund, as a moral justification for using a new and untried method. As a result there were many deaths in the early days of cardiac surgery and the rather dismal results were condemned loudly by established clinicians.

Kolff had developed his artificial kidney in Holland during the German occupation and when he sent one machine to Hammersmith it was used on patients with renal failure who had a chance of recovering normal kidney function. It was not used on patients with terminal renal failure, opinion was that these patients needed a kidney transplant not dialysis. Aird thought that renal transplantation was possible: Dempster did the experimental work in dogs and Shackman showed that it was feasible in patients. The first transplants were taken from relatives – a difficult moral decision for the relative, donor and surgeon – and this too evoked much criticism. In the U.S.A., renal dialysis was introduced as the method of choice of treatment for renal failure (although opinion has now confirmed that a transplant is better, cheaper and more certain) and in some ways Hammersmith would have received less caustic criticism if dialysis had been made the preliminary to transplantation. The problem of how to match donor and recipient for immunological compatibility was solved temporarily over lunch-time in 1963. All patients were medicated with a suppressive drug (Immuran, made by the Wellcome and supplied free to the U.S.A. for many years because it did not receive F.D.A. approval until much later) for 6 weeks. The Plastic Surgeon would then take a skin graft from the proposed donor (sometimes, but rarely, more than one) and apply this to the left forearm of the intended recipient: at the same time the recipient had an autograft of skin so that both grafts could be compared fairly and eliminate quirks of technique. The grafts were inspected and photographed and if the homograft survived intact for 6 weeks the renal transplant went ahead. The method was remarkably successful in predicting the outcome of the kidney graft (but, of course, only of one-way predictive value) and for the first 3 years was the sole method available. In 1966 the matching of antigens was introduced, which also facilitated the use of cadaver kidneys. Even so, one occasionally recognized a patient nearly 20 years later by the unusual skin grafts on the volar aspect of the left forearm even when the patient no longer remembered the reason for them (which had been carefully explained at the time) or the name of his surgeon (although printed on his bed-head during his stay in hospital). When criticism was levelled at transplants as late as 1976 it was easy to demonstrate that no patient thus treated had died because of his treatment over the previous 10 years: a denial that gave great satisfaction to the collector of records, but was simply not believed by the accuser.

CASE MIX

The distinction between training and education mentioned in previous chapters was highlighted even more in the clinical practice of the Hammersmith, where it was perfectly natural for any doctor to narrow down his area of clinical interest just to be able to study a single condition. For registrars in training this would not do, and in the late seventies various specialty boards of the Royal Colleges declined certification. As already noted, educating people is not done by instant fiat: it takes time and a variety of different processes of learning and teaching.

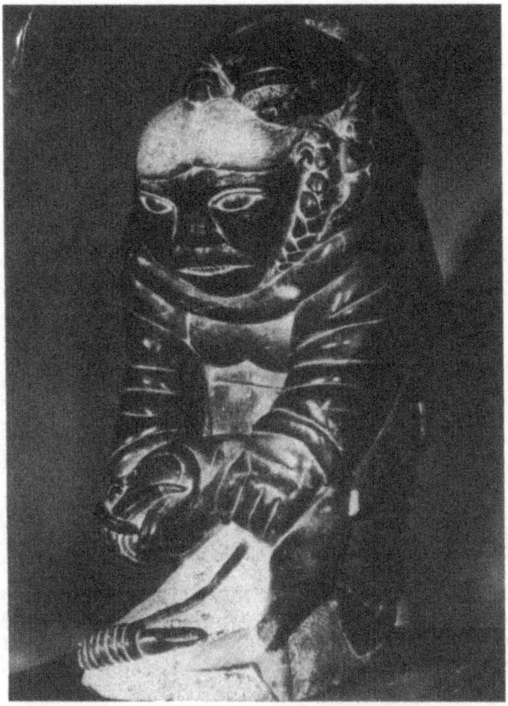

Figure 61 Close-up of the green soapstone Eskimo sculpture in the entrance hall of the Commonwealth Building, probably the largest in the U.K.: it shows an Eskimo woman fishing at a hole in the ice, a salmon at her feet, her papoose on her back holding a snow-goose

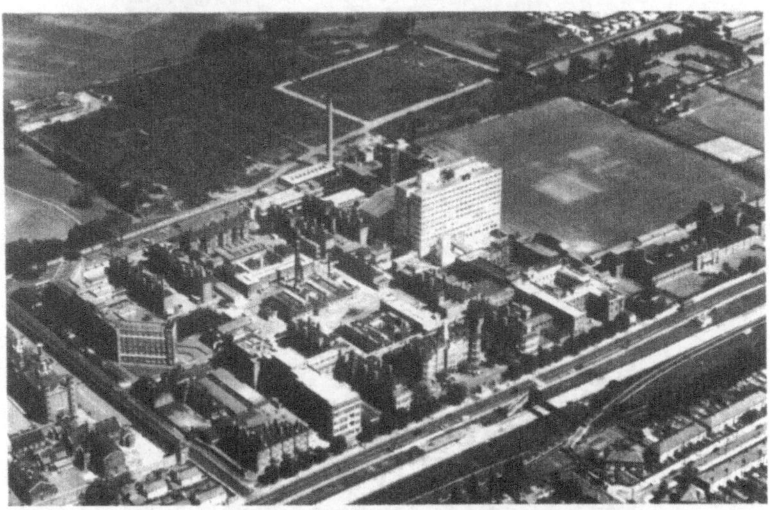

Figure 62 *c.* 1967. Aerial view of the site showing the Commonwealth Building, the large playing fields of the school next door, on which helicopters used to land, and the cleared Army Recruiting Depot (above)

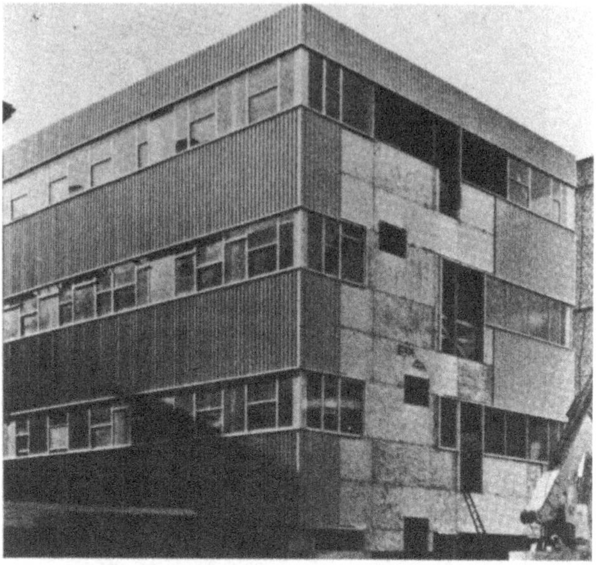

Figure 63 1969. The industrial-type building being completed between C and D blocks, for an intensive care unit, operating theatre, renal transplant unit, and special diet kitchen (this was built on the site of the original X-ray room and operating theatre of the Hammersmith Hospital of 1905)

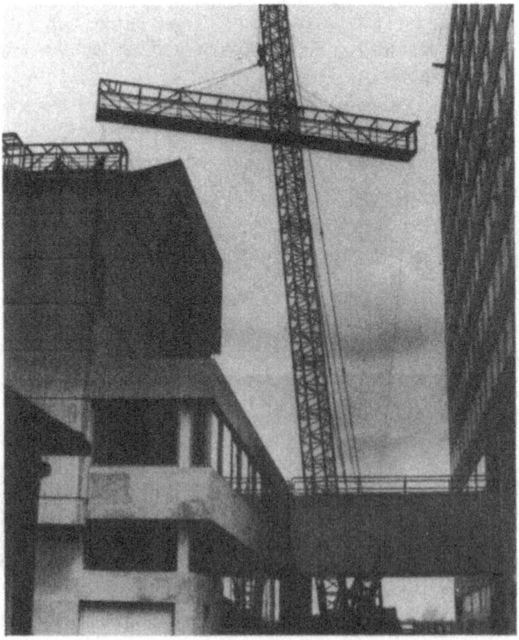

Figure 64 March 1969. The Aird Bridge being hoisted into position

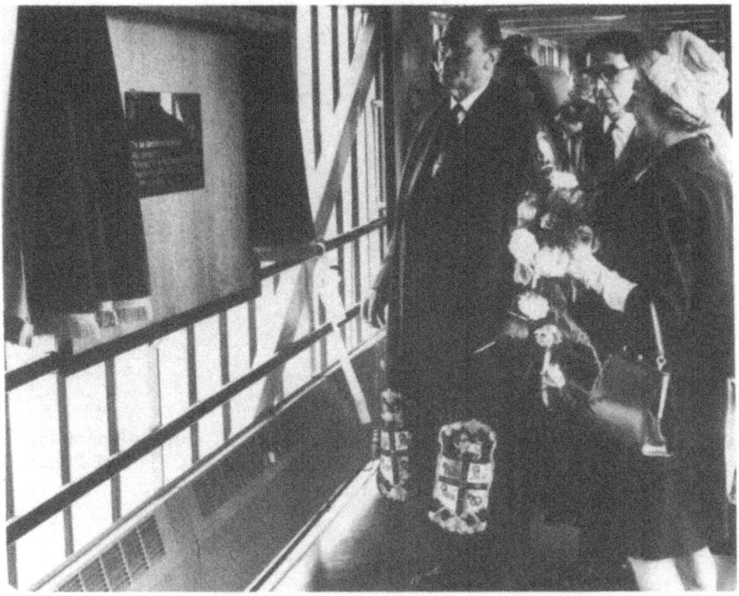

Figure 65 19 June 1969. The Aird Bridge opened officially by Professor Sir Hedley Atkins, President of the Royal College of Surgeons, with Lady Atkins. Professor Welbourn, Head of the Department of Surgery at the Royal Postgraduate Medical School is seen between them

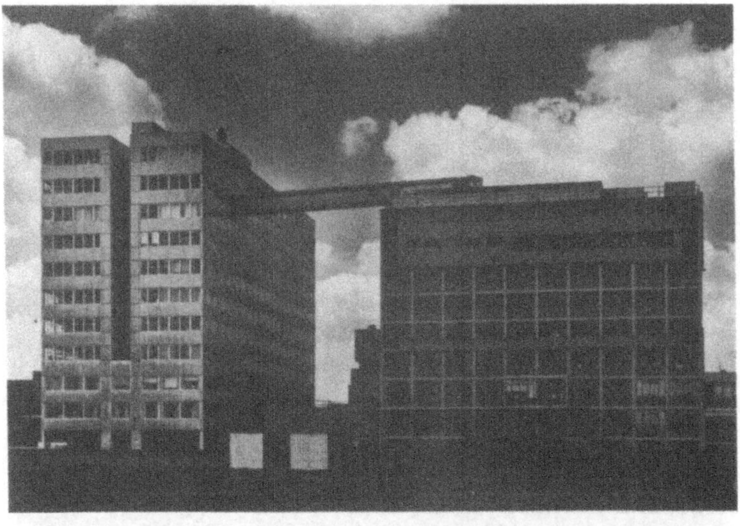

Figure 66 The Aird Bridge (not quite level) joining the Commonwealth Building (left) to the Surgical Research Laboratories in the Cyclotron Building (right) seen from the playing fields (note white cricket screens in foreground).

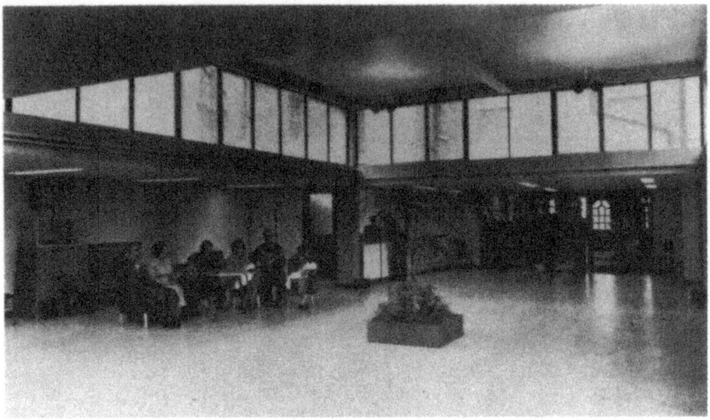

Figure 67 The front reception hall of the Hospital in 1957; the spacious appearance. Note, beneath the wall clock (left), the fish-tank and firebuckets. The Hall Porters, James and House, are standing at the front door

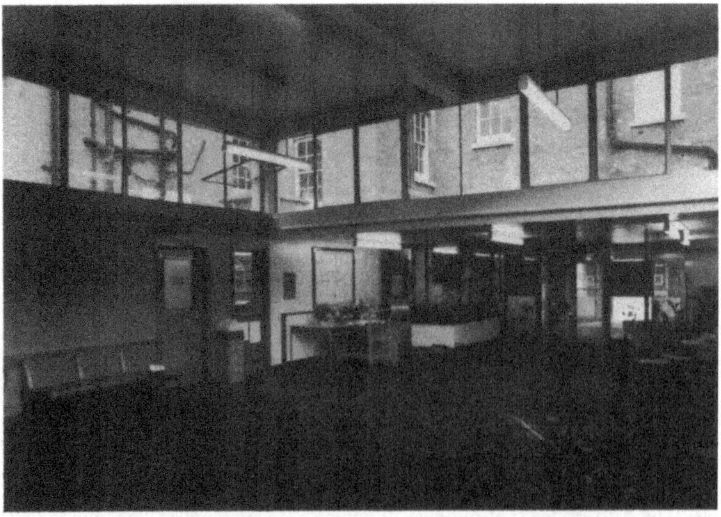

Figure 68 The same hall in 1984; the waiting area is half the size and there has been considerable in-filling by offices

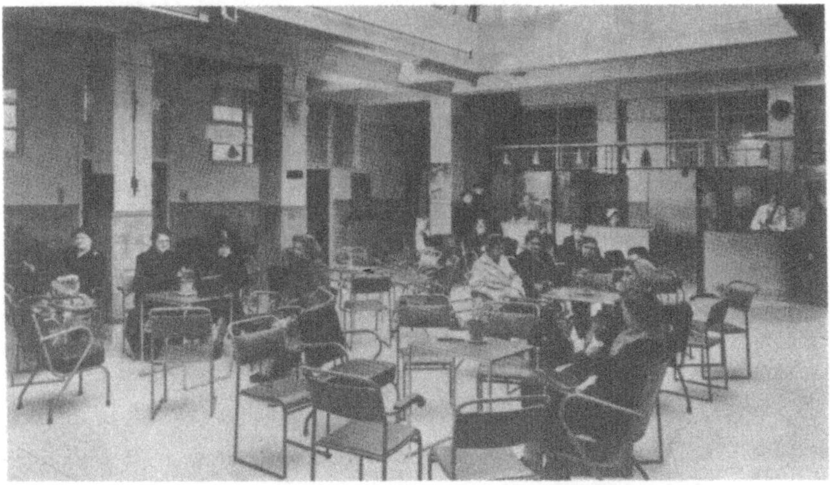

Figure 69 The Out-patient waiting area in 1955, virtually unchanged since 1935

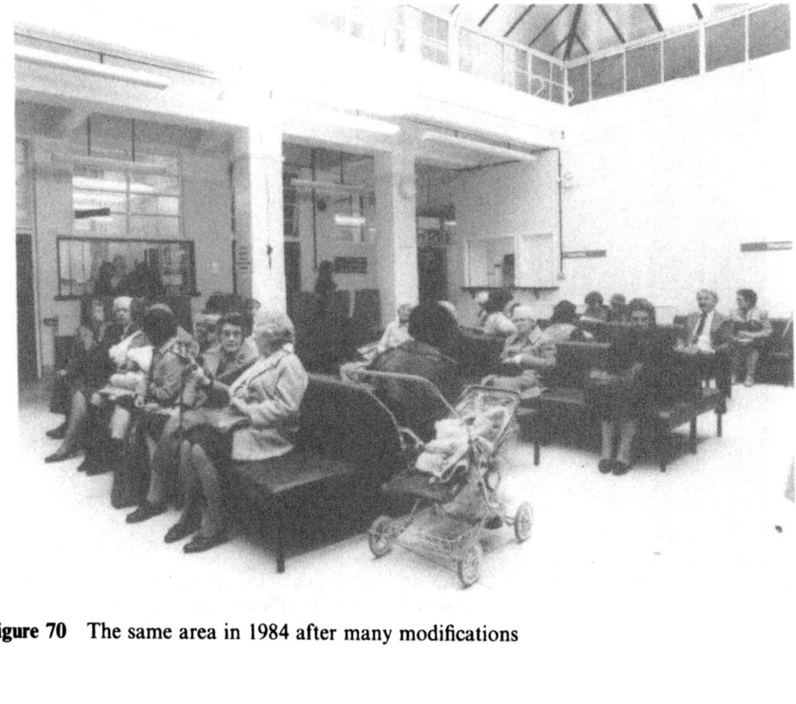

Figure 70 The same area in 1984 after many modifications

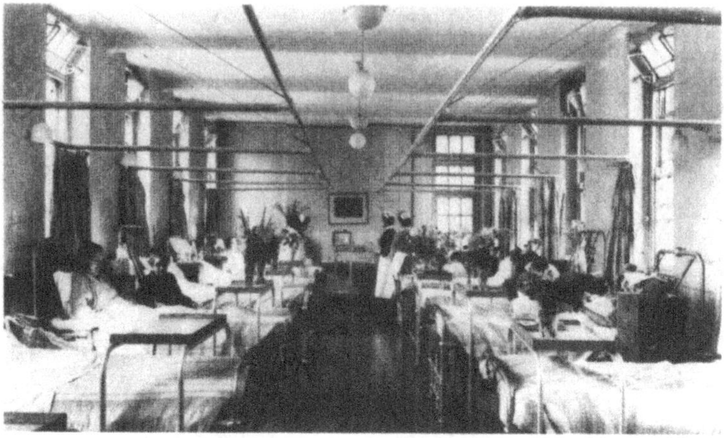

Figure 71 The first ward T.V. set, donated by the Friends of Hammersmith Hospital in 1958

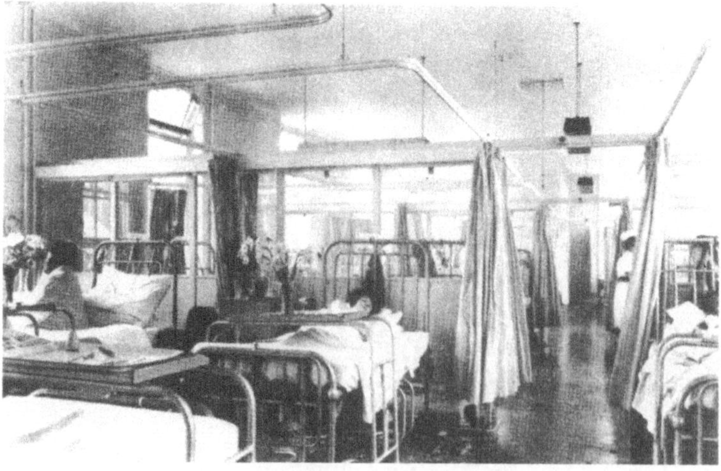

Figure 72 The same ward after modernisation in 1963: the cubicles separated by glass and metal panels made the ward more crowded and more difficult to observe all patients at a glance

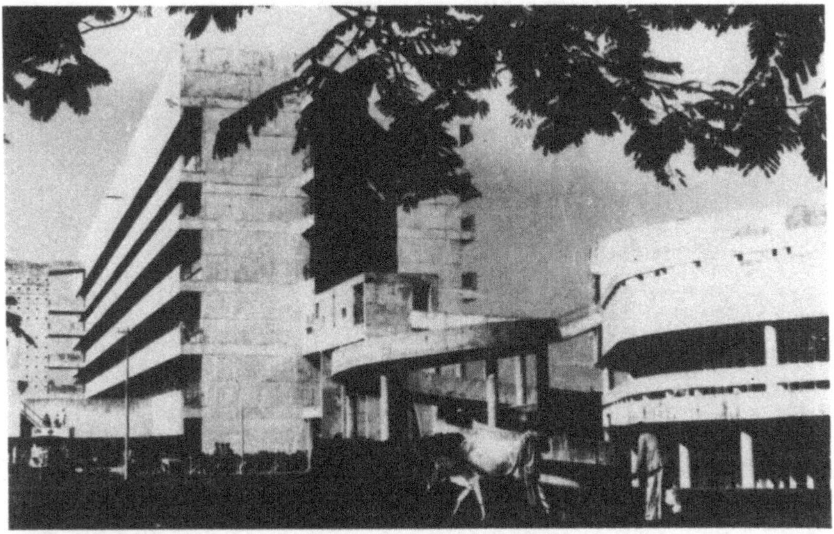

Figure 73 October 1972 at Chandigarh. Note the old and new

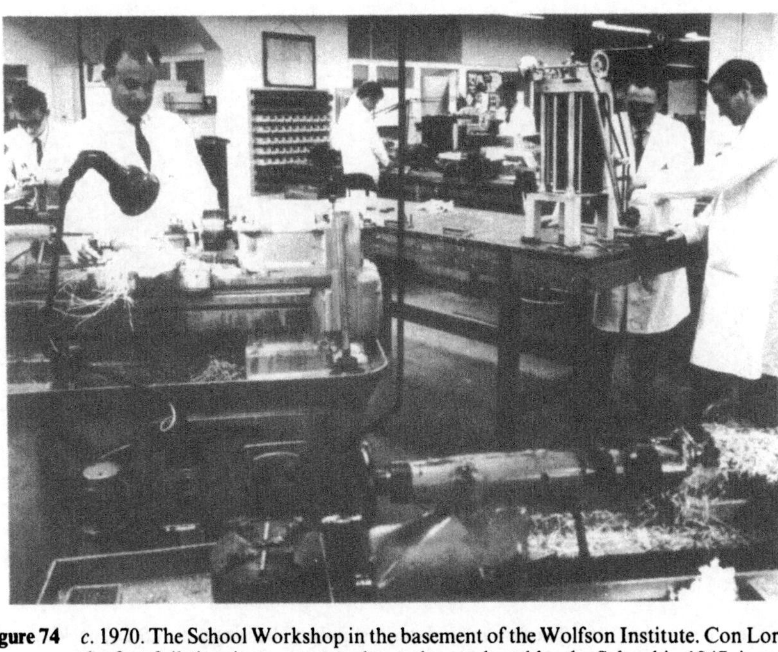

Figure 74 *c.* 1970. The School Workshop in the basement of the Wolfson Institute. Con Lordan, the first full-time instrument-maker to be employed by the School in 1947, is second from the right. The total area was about 500 m^2 and 20 people worked there

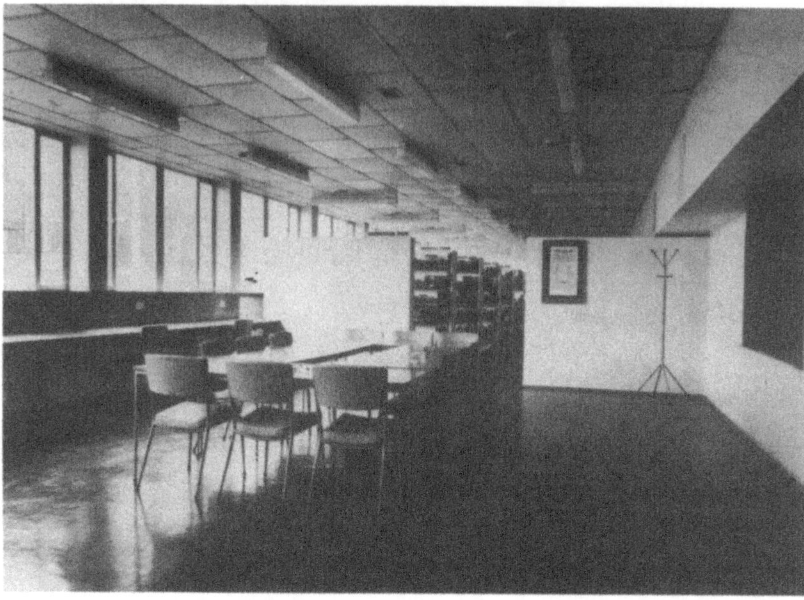

Figure 75 Conference rooms and museum (see beyond) on the third floor of the Commonwealth Building in 1967. Note the hat-stand (right) for white coats not hats, and the ubiquitous blackboard

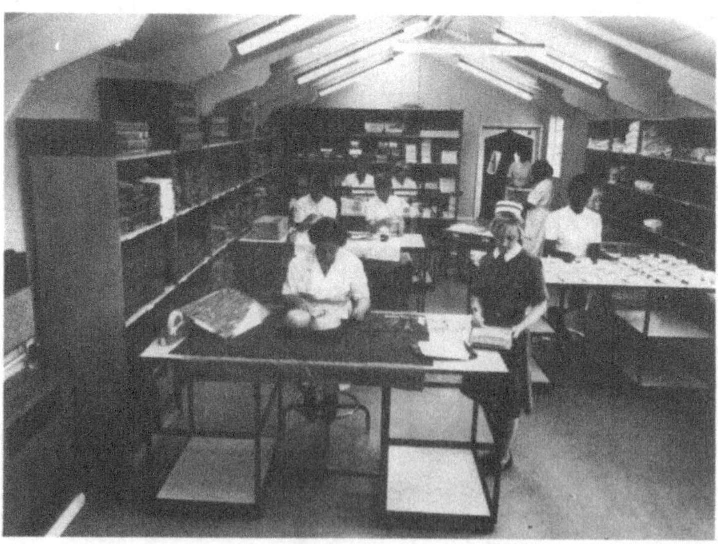

Figure 76 November 1967. The first 'central sterile supply of dressings' (C.S.S.D.) packing room in one of the wooden huts behind the Hospital corridor. The storage heater (lower left) was the sole supply of heat

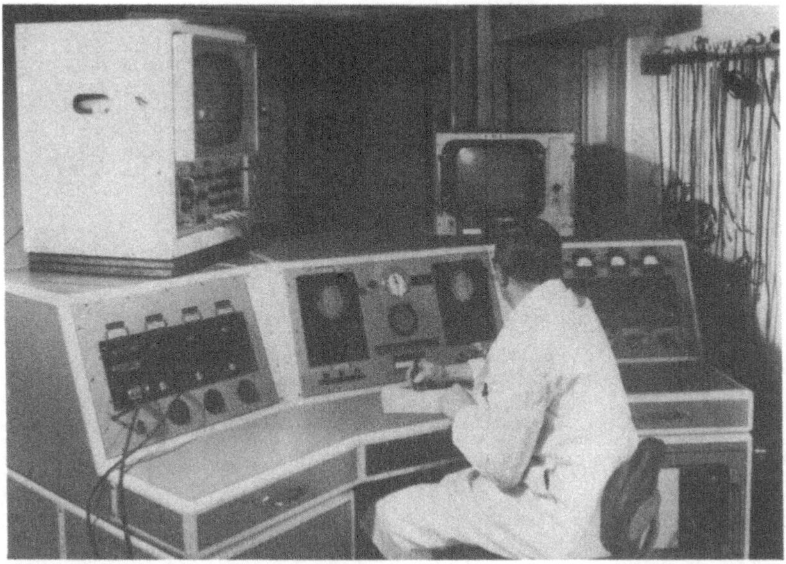

Figure 77 The monitoring room attached to the theatre for cardiac surgery (which can be seen through the window above the console. The television screen (right) showed a close-up of the operation, the camera being mounted in the theatre light. The technician could talk to the surgeon by microphone

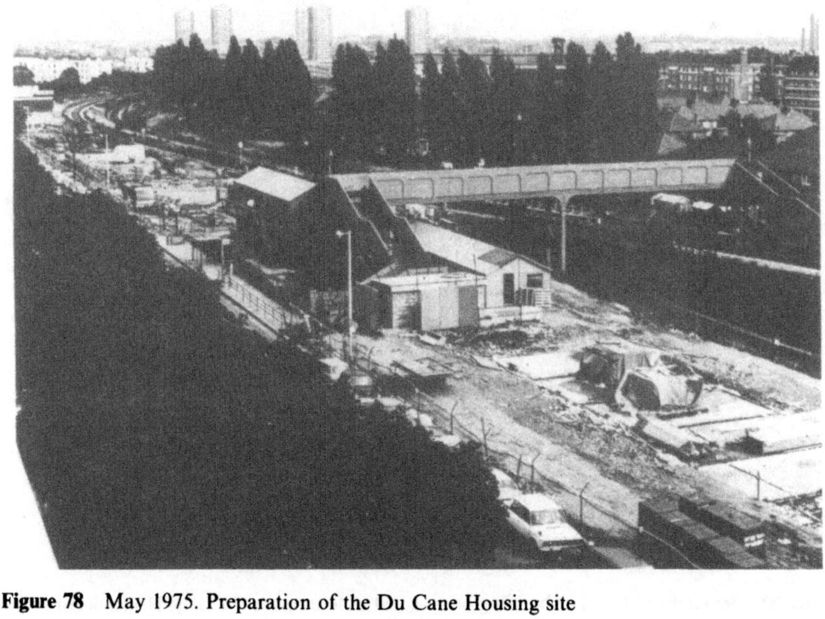

Figure 78 May 1975. Preparation of the Du Cane Housing site

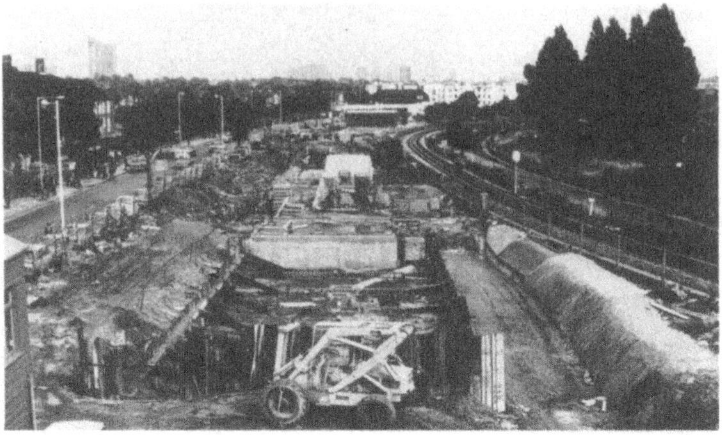

Figure 79 Another view of the Du Cane Housing site with foundations completed

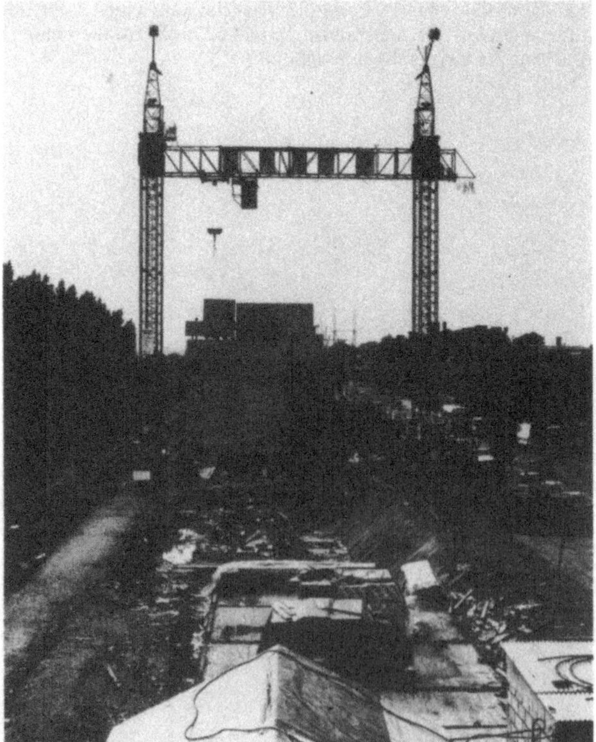

Figure 80 September 1975. The building block construction of the Du Cane Housing complex

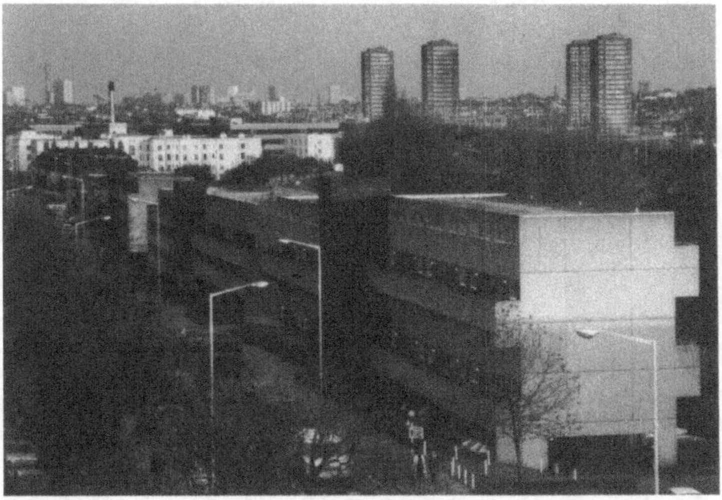

Figure 81 The Du Cane Housing 112 apartments in 1984

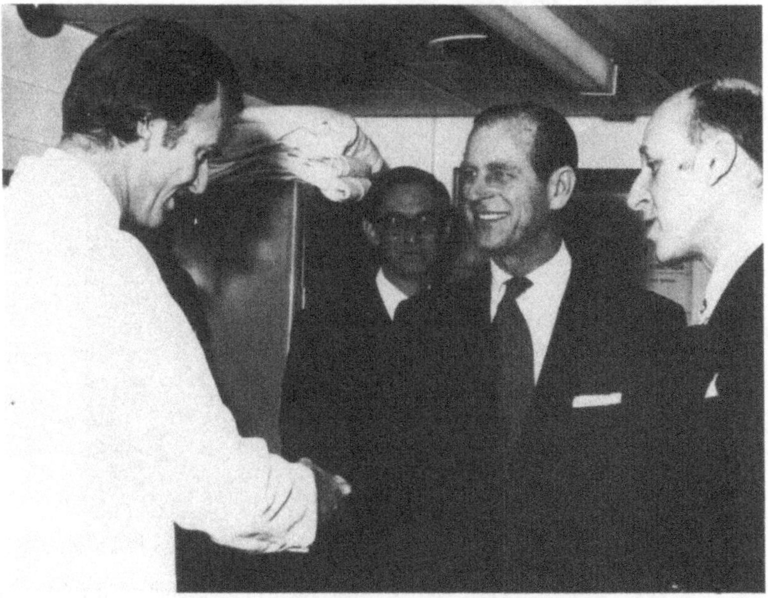

Figure 82 11 March 1976. The President, H.R.H. Prince Philip the Duke of Edinburgh, pays an informal visit to the School. Left to right: Professor Dollery, Professor Robson, H.R.H., the Dean Dr Malcolm Godfrey

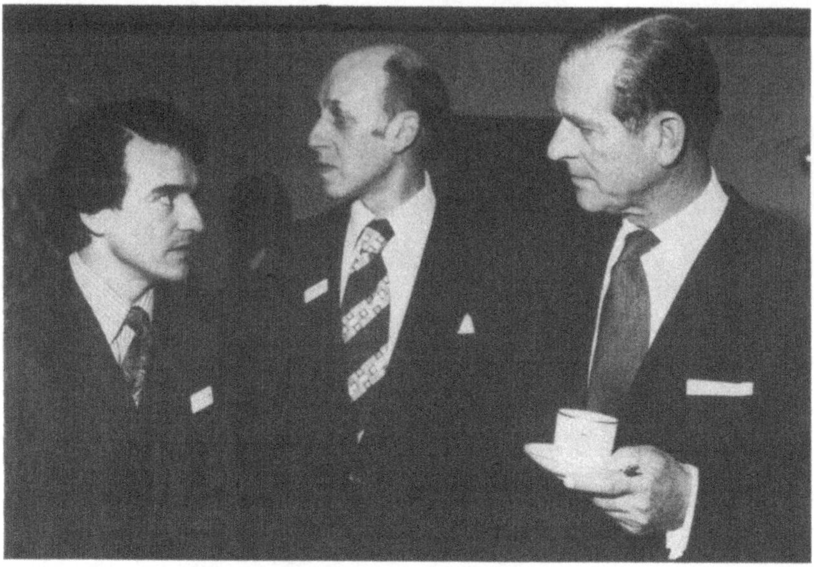

Figure 83 11 March 1976. Left to right: Dr Allison, the Dean, the Duke of Edinburgh (the then President of the School)

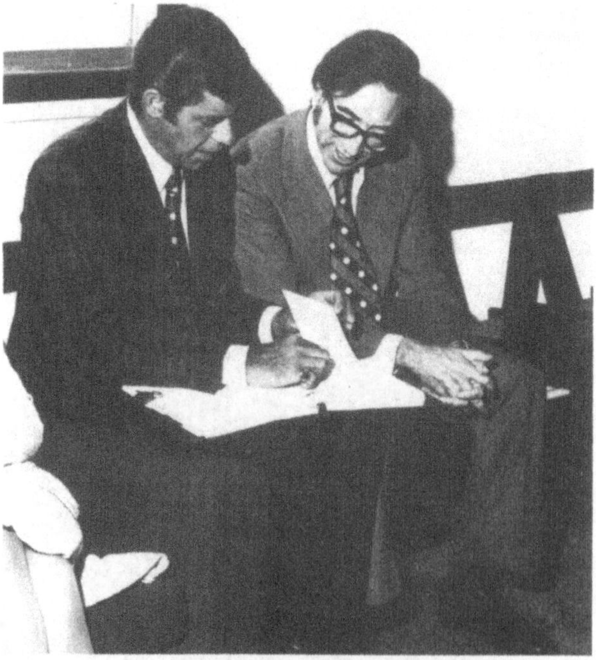

Figure 84 1975. Jerry Lewis with Professor Dubowitz at the opening of the Jerry Lewis Laboratories for research into muscular disorders. The American Muscular Dystrophy Association had awarded £125,000 (the first ever award outside the U.S.A.) for a suite of labs built on the roof of L block

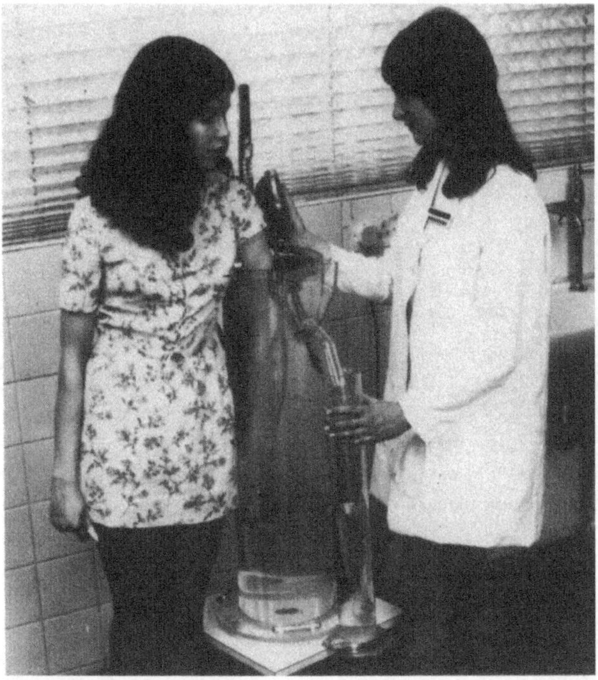

Figure 85 Simple research, measuring the arm volume with apparatus made on site, but note the miniskirts and how technicians had to shorten the hem of their white coats: *c.* 1970

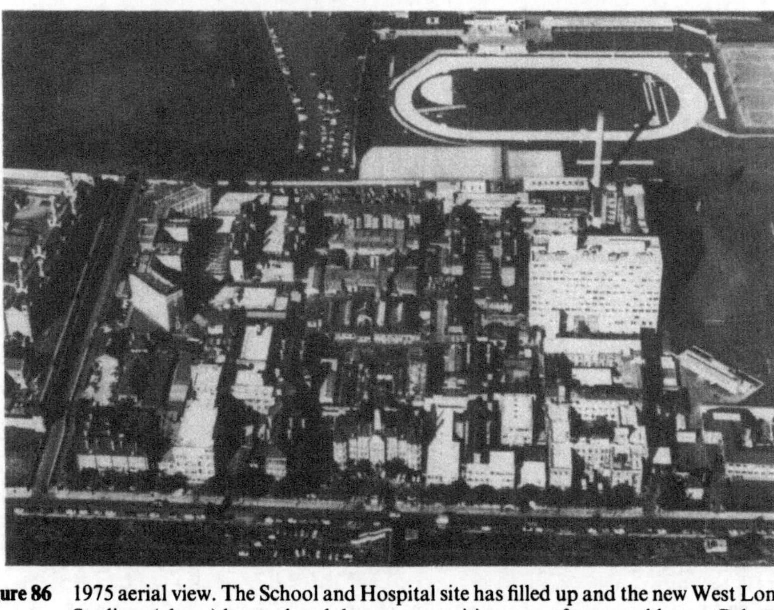

Figure 86 1975 aerial view. The School and Hospital site has filled up and the new West London Stadium (above) has replaced the army recruiting area of two world wars. Below, the Du Cane Housing complex is beginning to rise from the disused railway line

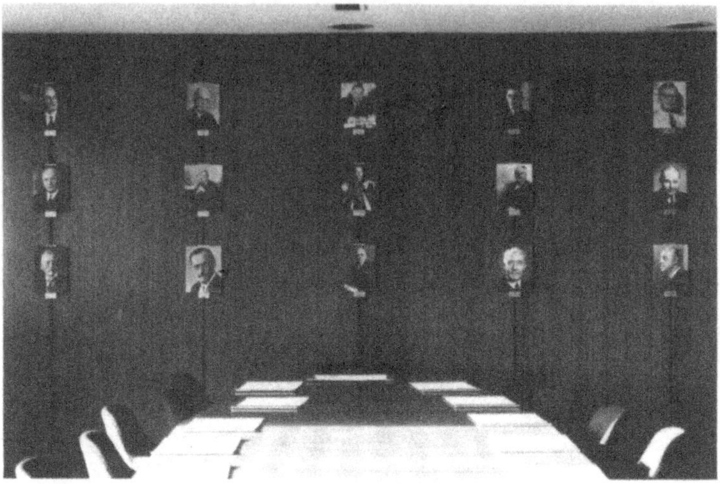

Figure 87 In memoriam: the wall of fame in the School Boardroom

Figure 88 In memoriam: donors to the School building inscribed on green marble on the first floor concourse of the Commonwealth Building linking the old School with the new

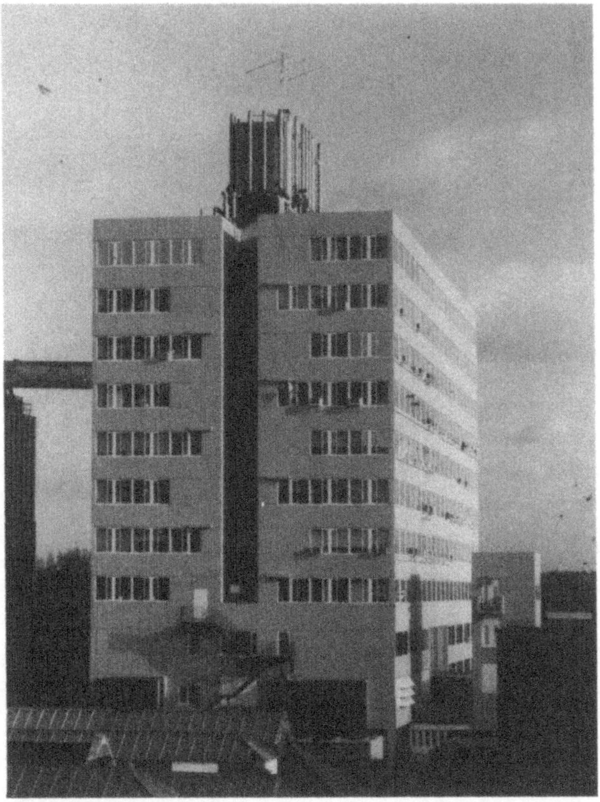

Figure 89 The 1984 School

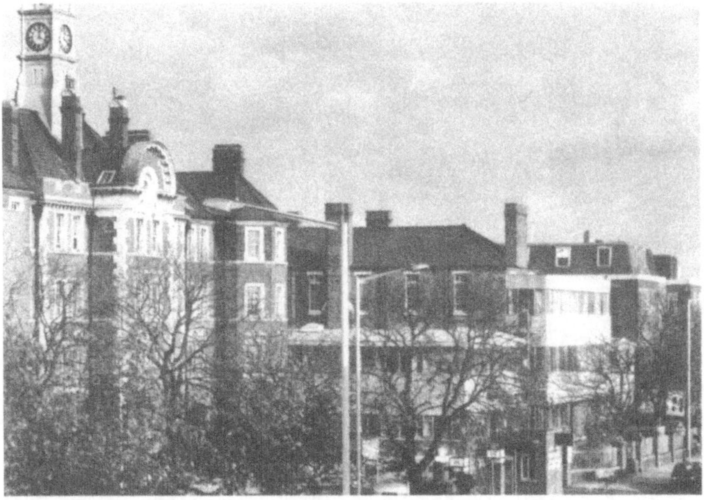

Figure 90 The 1984 Hospital

A variety must also be present in the 'case mix' of patients. As early as 1938 Grey Turner had written about surgery: 'It would be to the advantage of the unit to have a large proportion of the more ordinary type of case. The problems they present are of much interest to many of the students who state that they are never called to deal with the more complicated types of cases which naturally come to a hospital where the greater number of the patients are specially recommended.' In 1938 admissions to L.C.C. hospitals depended on the residence of the patient: those from the West end of Du Cane Road could come to Hammersmith, those from the other end could not. By special dispensation the Foundation Professors could admit patients referred to them personally, irrespective of address, and Sir Kay Menzies, Chief Medical Officer to the L.C.C., had promised that referrals from other hospitals to Hammersmith would be facilitated. The introduction of the N.H.S. Act in 1948 changed all that: there was complete freedom of the patient to go to the hospital of his choice and of his family doctor to refer him where he liked. The modern generation of patients do not always appreciate this liberalization of movement but officers in finance and administration of popular hospitals realize it too well.

The problem of 'case mix' of patients for higher training was to be a recurring complaint in all clinical departments for the next 40 years. Some were overwhelmed by their own fame and expertise in one particular disease or treatment, others because of a particular service: some had more patients than they could deal with, others less. The Founding Professors all had large and important textbooks to their names – this was the usual method of obtaining recognition in a particular field before the war – but none are in current use. The second generation of Professors tended to publish papers in scientific journals rather than textbooks. Ian Aird's book, *Companion to Surgical Studies*, in 1956, was unusual in many respects: it was the only textbook of surgery without illustrations, its 1200 pages were by a single author, and its contents were dictated to his secretary (Miss Matthews) and sent to the publishers without a single revision.

In the early days the quality of the students accepted was a matter of concern and this concern has returned in the past few years when the level of fees charge was increased drastically by government decree in 1979. In the 1937 annual report the Professor of Medicine, Francis Fraser, wrote: 'The students are for the most part candidates for higher degrees in medicine, such as the M.D. of the University or the Membership of the Royal College of Physicians, and are expected to work in the Department for three months or longer, during which time they act as clinical clerks on the wards. Only about half of the students work seriously as clinical clerks and so utilize the opportunities to best advantage. Some attend for too short a time to take an effective part in the ward work, and others are not able because of defects in their previous training to study advantageously by themselves.'

Fraser's complaint was completely negated 10 years later. The Second World War brought antibiotics, new surgical techniques, atomic medicine and such a spur to research for the benefit of patients that the Hammersmith seemed about to burst at the seams. Large numbers of very experienced doctors (old heads on young shoulders, a product of the battlefield) jostled for recognition and a job as the National Health Service began to shape the direction of British Medicine. The times called for a new kind of scientist–doctor, someone who combined the practice of medicine with a sound knowledge of science and an instinct for experimentation. Clinical research as we know it today – a kind of two-way exchange of ideas, information and experience between the laboratory and the patient's bedside – had started at Hammersmith in 1935 but never had the chance to blossom until after the war, and even then the rationing of space and materials deferred by a decade the progress that was to come.

All the Foundation Professors had indicated that it was an academic duty to experiment in treatment, to push techniques to the limit of knowledge, to take those risks that others were not prepared to take in pushing the frontiers of knowledge further than even visualized.

The war graduates accepted this philosophy and created clinical practice on the lines laid down by research and teaching: the practice of medicine changed dramatically and permanently. In clinical research, perhaps more than in any other field of human endeavour, one thing leads to another. Free choice of problems and free choice to follow leads disclosed by the solution of a first problem must be the privilege of the clinician. If he strikes a hot scent the means must be found to permit him to follow with vigour: to this end, the main function of a head of department is to facilitate funds, create posts, make room, try to understand and support the new methods. Recurrent Government fears that research was being duplicated, that the findings not implemented, or that the return on monies spent did not relate to the problems that needed to be solved, were rarely true at Hammersmith. The reverse was true: new techniques were introduced quickly.

Modern medicine is expensive medicine, when current knowledge is applied and especially to patients with intractable complaints. In 1983 the budget[94] for the 500 or so beds in use at Hammersmith Hospital was £28 million: for St Mary's, Praed Street of 439 beds £22 million, the West Middlesex University Hospital (a new breed of recognition) of 814 beds, £21 million: even for the 817 beds at M.R.C. Clinical Research Unit (a mix of M.R.C. and N.H.S. services quite different from the Hammersmith structure) £25 million. Yet there was no real difference between the kind of medicine required at an undergraduate teaching hospital, district general hospital, or postgraduate teaching centre as far as the patient was concerned. Or was there?

OUT-PATIENTS

At the time that the School was being built, the London County Council improved the accommodation in Hammersmith Hospital by adding new

Table 5 Out-patients, 1953–1983

	1953	*1963*	*1973*	*1983*
New out-patients	23,553	23,525	24,719	18,056
Total out-patients	89,875	114,077	123,904	116,364
Percentage new of total	26%	21%	20%	15%

operating theatres, a new X-ray department, and creating an out-patient department. For the last building, on the ground floor at the front of the hospital, it was estimated that clinic rooms were needed to allow about 70 patients to be seen daily – hospital medicine was practised as a 6-day week in 1935 – a maximum total of 20,000 patients a year. The figure was easily exceeded soon after the war as the statistics in Table 5 show.[95]

In 1983, on a 5-day week, an average of 447 patients were seen daily in what was virtually the same building as 1935. The total number of patients had increased by 30% since 1953 but the number of new referrals had remained about the same (the drop in 1983 may be significant). The explanation for the contrasting figures, proposed in the early seventies (when the N.H.S. was seriously looking for economies) was that consultants refused to discharge their clinic patients back to the care of the patient's general practitioner. In spite of a drive to get rid of 'follow-ups' the number continued to rise. The more likely explanation was that medical practice had changed in 30 years (1953–1983) in three ways. First, there had been an increasing use of out-patient facilities rather than in-patient admission for investigative procedures, particularly in radiology, endoscopy, blood and chemical analyses. Second, there had been an increase in out-patient rather than in-patient treatment for chest infections, heart disease, children, anti-cancer therapy, and day-care surgery (20–30% of all surgery at Hammersmith). Third, an increase in controlled trials of new drugs – and a large increase in new therapeutic agents limited to hospital use only until assessed – which often necessitated regular surveillance of the patient by clinical inspection and frequent biochemical or haematological estimations (in 1963 there were on an average day about 30 trials in progress, by 1983 double that).

IN-PATIENTS

There were equally noticeable changes when one examines in-patient statistics (Table 6).

The fall in the average length of stay in hospital by half of what it was 30 years ago is in line with the national average, and is attributed to im-

Table 6 In-patients, 1953–1983

	1953	*1963*	*1973*	*1983*
Beds available	653	659	624	548
Beds occupied	565	571	501	453
Percentage occupied	86%	86%	80%	83%
Number of in-patients	11,516	13,674	15,908	18,249
Average length of stay in days	17.8	15.3	12.4	9.1

provements in medical management. The decrease in the number of available beds by 16% is also in line with the national trend. There has, however, been a 58% increase in the number of in-patients: partly due to treatment not available 30 years ago (such as most of cardiac surgery, major liver surgery, management of hypertension and renal failure, and many others), an older population with greater expectations of recovery from intractable conditions, and a significant occurrence of iatrogenic disease.

CLINICAL CO-OPERATION

Demarcation lines between clinical departments are as deeply dividing as they are between labour unions. Some disappear with time, others when advantages are seen to accrue to both sides (such as the creation of the Division of Cardiology – medicine and surgery – in 1976), some when their function has served its purpose, others when positive attempts are made to demolish them for a new vision; such visionaries collated medicine and surgery in heart, intestinal, and renal disease, but with no guarantee of permanent union, just the fecundity of the aggregation of intellects and the stimulating effects of intellectual attrition. Two minds can focus on a single problem, uniting their labours in its solution, when such co-operation is truly spontaneous: when imposed upon them by someone seeking to compel the investigation of a particular subject there is apt to be sterility. The words of Alan Gregg of the Rockefeller Foundation are apposite: 'I suggest that something extraordinary precious comes out of the close but entirely free association of really superior people. To this emergent quality I give the name 'the heritage of excellence', mostly because it lasts so long and because it never comes from, nor appeals to, mediocrities. . . .'

Medicine differs from most other professions where one can hold a degree in a subject, boast and never have to practise. Medicine has to be practised to be anything, and reputations depend on the quality of that practice, not the quantity. Hammersmith had a large overseas practice from which the School and the N.H.S. benefited: patients came because they recognized quality and needed something not available in their own country. Ironically, the Hammersmith had few accommodations for those who wished to enter as private patients. There was no private wing, only a limited number of single rooms attached to main wards, and no match for the growing demand. In the sixties the number of beds delegated as 'private' – and many were in main wards yet, disgracefully, patients were charged top rates for inferior accommodation – was 20, to be reduced to 18 in the seventies. The numbers were often exceeded, not from any desire for monetary gain by individual physicians or surgeons but because most patients were from abroad and designated 'private' because they were not entitled to benefit from the 'free' N.H.S. Relations between the D.H.S.S. and Hammersmith became increasingly acrimonious when patients landed at London Airport for admission to hospital and clearly were too ill to return to their homeland.

In spite of the fact that private patients at Hammersmith were accommodated in inferior quarters with none of the amenities expected in an advanced country (such as private telephone, television, bathroom en suite, security for personal belongings, secretarial service for commercial needs) and often little privacy, yet they continued to come, and their presence made possible the perpetuations of individual departmental R&D funds (by 1984, a total sum approaching £1 million and hence a major economic factor in the runnng of the School). Statistics for the numbers of private patients seen during a decade or more are not available, but from 1978 to 1983 (a 6-year period) a total of 11,958 patients were seen in consultation of which 5046 (42%) were new referrals. The number of new patients annually had risen slowly from 672 to 995 – and there were 543 in the first 6 months of 1984 – but these almost certainly represent less than 50% capacity. The amount in lost fees and lost opportunities over the past 30 years can be considered a large sum both for School and N.H.S.

OVERSEAS TRAVEL

One of the more obvious effects of Hammersmith's obsession with research and teaching as instruments of good clinical practice was travel abroad. All the Foundation Professors travelled extensively but the post-war traveller was different. He did three things. First, he got away from a closed environment and saw the world as it was beyond his lab. and the hospital gates. Second, he spread the gospel of good medical practice, giving his own results (which were often unique and impressive) and how research in the subject was going. Third, he absorbed, observed and interpreted other people's problems: he brought them back as suitable research projects for his juniors. The system worked. The system worked so well that humorous stories were generated, questions asked, hackles raised, and a moratorium placed on overseas travel during term-time, but all to no avail. Hammersmith was in the import and export business, the whole affair became respectable, and for the past 20 years the travels abroad of members have been recorded in the annual reports of the School. They read like a Baedeker Guide and tell the reader where the new in medicine is being developed. In 1983 over 145 members of staff lectured in 38 countries, some more than once in the same country: the majority of this export traffic was to Europe (37%) rather than with the U.S.A. (25%), a complete reversal of the pattern of 10 years earlier. Sixty-eight visitors, mainly Professors, came to see the Hammersmith from 25 countries. But already in 1983 many departments no longer bothered to record visits of staff to lecture abroad, preferring to declare the results of clinical research work completed on site or in collaboration with other centres. Foreign travel costs money. Some funds were set up when the School first started, specifically to aid travel (and thus were novel), but the great majority are of recent origin and stem from private patients' fees allocated to departments.

There can be little doubt that foreign travel by staff did two things for School and Hospital more effectively, and probably more cheaply, than any advertising campaign: it made the name of the Hammersmith well known across the world, and fired the imagination of bright young men and women (often the best brains in their country) to come and work here. Some of the evangelists worked with a fervour comparable to that of the early Christians and drew adverse comment on their frequent and prolonged absences from their place of work, but there is little doubt that travel brought incalculable advantages to School, Hospital and staff. Hammersmith had to encourage the entrepreneur of clinical practice as much as it had to encourage the entrepreneur in research. Every entrepreneur is a kind of outsider with a detachment which enables him to see and exploit opportunities: in commercial life nomadic instincts and risk-taking are usually associated with the term. Hammersmith never pretended to give staff a sense of community or security but recognized that foreign travel broadened contacts – in some cases could narrow them fruitfully by visits to other clinicians in the same field – and was cost-effective.

THE CHANGING SERVICE

There have always been gaps in the clinical services offered, and a lack of development in others, for a variety of reasons. In recent years there has been a change in the age of the population and the increasing importance of chronic and degenerative diseases has posed new problems for the N.H.S. The growing proportion of elderly, mentally and physically disabled in the country had been neglected. At Hammersmith the post of part-time lecturer (Geriatrics) had been created to look after a population of unvarying patients in 20 beds in one ward, for care not cure, a type of custodial management at variance with the general attitude at the Hammersmith. The patients were old ladies who could no longer look after themselves. The first holder was Lord Amulree in 1952 (he was a Consultant Physician at University College Hospital 1949–1966, and resigned from Hammersmith in 1954 to become Liberal Whip in the House of Lords), who was followed by Gilliland. By the time the latter retired, in 1974, there had been a shift in the population of England and Wales (and in the whole of the Western world for that matter) which had serious implications for the future of the School and the N.H.S. The figures to note (as 20-year differences)[96] are as shown in Table 7.

Table 7 Population figures, England and Wales, 1961 and 1980

	1961 (*millions*)	*1980* (*millions*)	*Increase* (%)
Total population	46.1	49.6	8
Over 65 years	5.5	7.5	36
Over 75 years	2	3	50

It was already known that people over 75 use about four times more of the resources of the N.H.S. than any other group of patients, and for acute general hospitals this could mean that an unacceptably high proportion of beds in future would be devoted to the care of the elderly. The pressure for some kind of solution was national. Hammersmith created an academic Chair in Geriatric Medicine in 1979 (Hodkinson the first incumbent) with the expectation that research into the biological process of ageing and diseases of old age will be as productive as the research conducted in other fields.

14

The Years of Uncertainty and Unrest (1970–1978)

The Heath Government of 1970–1974 had one radical aim: to break with the State interventionist and consensus welfare policies of previous Labour and Conservative governments, an aim that was to resurface with the Thatcher Government of 1979. Government expenditure would be cut, individuals would have fatter pay packets, commercial enterprises would not be bailed out at the taxpayer's expense, inflation would be reduced, people were to become more responsible and self-sufficient. Those who could not cope would qualify for social benefits and thereby help was to be concentrated where it was needed most. Unfortunately this simplistic policy did not work out at the time, and for many reasons. Major reforms were passed by Parliament and put into effect: in 1971 the Industrial Relations Bill was implemented in August and was to sour relations for the remainder of the decade even after it was rescinded in 1974 (and without any evidence whether such legislation was workable). The Local Government Act, evolved by the Redcliffe-Maud Committee, was later to create arguments between Hammersmith and the Local Authority about co-terminosity of medical services in the reorganized N.H.S. and of the kind that had occurred in 1935 when the School was founded.

THE ROYAL COMMISSION

The N.H.S. reorganization introduced in 1973 by Sir Keith Joseph as Minister of Health and implemented by the Labour Government of the following year, adopted a 'managerial approach' to the N.H.S. hospitals which were to be run by Area Health Authorities responsible to the Minister, and General Practitioner Services run by Executive Councils also responsible to the Minister (it is interesting that the Griffiths' Report,[97] implemented by Norman Fowler in 1984, reinforced the same belief in an industrial-type 'management' with more control by Parliament). The Royal Commission on the National Health Service (Chairman, Sir Alex Merrison[98]) was set up 2 years later: 'To consider in the interest both of the patients and those who work in the National Health Service the best use and management of the financial and manpower resources of the National Health Service.' The terms of reference were pretty vague, but over 1000 items of written opinion and fact were submitted to the Royal Commission: the commonest mentioned the structure of the N.H.S. and only 10 were about waiting lists. There was general concern about the proportionate allocations of resources between 'cure' and 'care', a debate that continues today.

Both the School and the Committee of Vice-Chancellors and Principals submitted written documents. Both pointed to the lack of clarity with which the respective duties and functions of authorities and officers in the new structure had been defined, the lack of responsibility for medical education, the lack of an effective university voice in management at the area and regional levels (where staffing of clinical departments is determined): 'The three level structure inevitably imposes a strain in relations to the distribution of resources for medical education and adds to the delay and complexity in obtaining decisions.' To have to engage with the N.H.S. at three levels in place of the single level enjoyed by the Board of Governors was particularly frustrating for Hammersmith; a line of communication which had served well since 1935 was now destroyed. For those at the School this was a new experience which no one really accepted.

The University of London hammered home its message, with little effect: 'the interplay of research, teaching and patient care is fundamental and needs to be appreciated. They are inseparable. Research leads to better patient care (the Goodenough Report had said the same in 1944). Much of the necessary information for research is derived from the care of many patients. Teaching becomes unrealistic if it is divorced from patient care and becomes ossified to the point of danger if it is divorced from research.' This was very much the Hammersmith line in its demand for adequate finance in university hospitals. The Expenditure Committee of the Department of Education and Science, in 1976, had proclaimed that 'postgraduate education should be shaped not by student demand alone, but principally by the needs of the economy and of society as a whole'. The School accepted this, whatever it really meant, even though historically it was the far-sighted individuals who shaped events (and found the money) and not society, which did not have that kind of imagination: the trouble was that society accepted the fruits of research, but was rather reluctant to pay for them (which is understandable). The School argued that in general the function of medical schools and research institutes must be to generate new knowledge in medical science and to make its benefits available in medical practice: in other words, to build bridges between the molecule on the one hand and the community on the other.

One of the main recommendations of the previous Royal Commission on Medical Education 1965–1968 (Chairman, Lord Todd[99]) was that 'Postgraduate education should be a joint responsibility of the universities, the professional colleges, and the Health Departments, leading to an agreed pattern of professional training for all specialists (including general practice) linked to a new hospital career structure which may help to eliminate many present frustrations.' From this stemmed the Boards of Accreditation in various specialties, organized and conducted by the Royal Colleges (of Surgeons, Physicians, Obstetrics and Gynaecology, and more recently General Practice) but there had not been the same level of support from the Department of Health nor separate funding for 'in service' education. To some extent this deficiency may have been rectified when the National Health Service Training Authority was made a Special Health Authority by the 1982 reorganization. On the whole the School remained unconvinced that education (the reason for doing things) would be linked to training (the technical ability to do things), and the basic philosophy of the school was about education and learning and reasoning.

OUTCOMES

There were two outcomes from the Royal Commission. The first was the Report on the Working Party appointed by the Vice-Chancellor to enquire into the Postgraduate Medical Institutes of the University of London (the Morris Report[100]) which was mainly about the future of the Federation: to dissolve it or not? The idea of amalgamating undergraduate and postgraduate schools was unacceptable to Hammersmith, which pointed out that the main responsibility of undergraduate schools was to provide medical students with a knowledge of the scientific basis of medicine and to equip them with the skills which will enable them to practise, initially under supervision and subsequently independently. Postgraduate schools must greatly extend the process of independence and interdependence, and in particular should encourage a critical appraisal of newly won knowledge which may be of uncertain value. An active involvement by students in relevant research is therefore a cornerstone of postgraduate education. The Hammersmith was not constrained by the requirement (of the General Medical Council) to teach a basic curriculum and so was able to teach specialist courses and provide research training. The Morris Report did not know what to do with those centres known and respected world-wide for the quality of medical work, such as Moorfields Eye Hospital and the Hospital for Nervous Diseases which had been practising successfully before the Federation of 1947: they became Special Health Authorities in the 1982 reorganization.

The second outcome was the Resource Allocation Working Party (R.A.W.P.) of the N.H.S. in 1975, to 'Transfer resources from the so-called better provided Regional Health Authorities to those parts of the country where health resources are in even shorter supply.' This was a direct threat to the levels of junior staffing at Hammersmith. In October 1977 Professor Le Quesne's[101] committee reported to the Secretary of State on the disastrous effect reallocation was having on London medical schools, but with little effect. The R.A.W.P. formula was savaged in the medical press, both before and after implementation, but it had effectively set South against North and 10 years later the final result has still to be declared.

Then came the energy crisis. First, because of a resurgence of the war between Egypt and Israel, oil production from the Arab states was reduced by 5% in October 1973 and a further 5% each month until a full settlement was reached for Israel to withdraw from the occupied Arab lands. Second, for Britain, a coal miner's strike resulting in the 3-day week in January 1974 and a General Election in February. The Wilson Labour Government was a minority party so that a further election was held in October when a working majority was obtained. The energy problem did not lose its threat until 1978 when British North Sea oil and natural gas were landed in reasonable quantities and prospects seem good for self-sufficiency in the eighties.

THE SCHOOL'S FUTURE

Seen against this background the future of the School in the seventies always appeared grim. First, there was the quinquennial submission. The major portion of the School's income came very properly from Government money and the route by which it arrived was from the Treasury to the University Grants Committee and then as a block grant to the University of London on to the British Postgraduate Medical Federation and finally to the School. Unfortunately money bags diminish as they travel. Every 5 years there was a review of the School's position, to consider the policy for the coming quinquennium and to propose a budget. The University Grants Medical Committee visited on 27 January 1970 and debated the 5-year period to begin in 1972. The School had grown and developed in the last 5 years more than ever before: there had been greater clinical demands, an expansion in postgraduate teaching, and an increase in research. Although patients had not increased in number their referral for conditions of complexity had, student numbers had increased, and the number of published papers had nearly doubled during the same period.

Money is indispensable for excellence and the School asked for a modest 3% increase in budget, yet the U.G.C. would not agree to any budget ahead of time. But the School was already committed, as it had been in the sixties by the opening of the new Experimental Surgical Unit (E.S.U.) in the M.R.C. Cyclotron Building and the demand to take over the heart–lung project (Melrose and Bentall) and the kidney transplant team (Dempster and Shackman) and all their revenue consequences.

No one seemed to appreciate that large new buildings attracted large new staff and tended to run into debt, as had occurred regularly in the N.H.S. when new hospitals were opened. There were earlier indications of financial troubles to come – the failure of the University to grant all 'equipment monies' according to the Pater[102] formula, entitled by the School for its new building – but no one took heed because no one wished to face the possibility of restrictions on medical progress. Instead there was an increase in applicants for research grants to provide technicians – now becoming known as medical laboratory scientific officers (M.L.S.O.) – to fill the bench space available and so fulfil the ambitions of those who wanted bigger and better labs. The number of grants increased from 139 in 1970 to 164 in 1978 but their total value rose from £518,506 to £2.16 million (yet inflation had decreased their real value by about half).

By 1975 the quinquennial system had been abandoned in favour of a system of 'cash limits' which made forward planning almost impossible. In that year the revenue grant was £1.464 million and the School had a deficit of £25,000. All new appointments were stopped. When the U.G.C. Medical Subcommittee visited in April, staff were interviewed in groups, this time by subject and not by seniority as previously in the early sixties. Between 1970 and 1975 the Hammersmith had provided 26 Professors (11 for the U.K.), 29 Readers and Senior Lecturers (21 for the U.K.), 20 postgraduates had been appointed to consultant posts in British teaching hospitals and 13 to similar posts overseas. The subcommittee was impressed. There was the promise of a new quinquennium in 2 years' time (1977–1982) but with inflation at 20% the revenue was unlikely to be enough to maintain current academic activity, let alone two new developments proposed (of psychiatry in general practice, and geriatric medicine), or to take over two units supported entirely by soft money grants (immunology and endocrinology).

The importance of the university quinquennial system of financing the School must be understood as the major opportunity for strategic planning. Hammersmith was quite prepared to solve pressing problems rather than develop long-run strategies by avoiding planning where plans depended on predictions of uncertain future events – the N.H.S. had done this for years, as the science of 'muddling through' – but not for major research directives: for these a quinquennial budget was mandatory. Planning is always an attempt to shape the future, by deciding where one wants to be at a fixed time and how to provide the resources needed to get there. Even Churchill had said: 'It is wise to plan ahead but difficult to look further than you can see', which sums up the problem. The future is always obscure but that does not obviate the need to plan: the main advantage of long-range corporate planning, even when it is based on fallible assumptions, is that it gives everyone a sense of direction, a purpose in life, and an idea of the resources needed for the future. Unrealistic planning can be avoided if the planning is limited to a period over which it is possible to forecast trends with fair accuracy, and to update plans regularly when conditions change. The period of planning agreed by universities was 5 years, a not unreasonable length of time.

But the School had already initiated six new units: a Department of Clinical Pharmacology (a very fast-growing research unit supported generously by the Medical Research Council, the Wellcome Foundation and many project research grants) set up by Dollery a good 10 years before the U.S.A. woke up to the idea that a specialty knowledge of the drugs that doctors prescribed daily was needed; a Department of Virology (made possible by Action for the Crippled Child); a Department of Immunology supported by the J. Pomeraniac Charitable Trust; an M.R.C. Leukaemia Therapy Unit (the Hospital was building the clinic rooms, but preferred to label them the 'Anaemia Unit'); a Unit of Statistics linked to the London School of Hygiene and Tropical Medicine (the main base) and St Mary's Hospital Medical School by money from the Leverhulme Trust; and recognition of the M.R.C. Haemolytic Mechanisms Group. The Hospital also started a four-floor industrial-type building for a new Intensive Care Unit, Renal Transplant Unit, and shell of an operating theatre with a corridor of laboratories, and a central sterilizing unit on the ground floor. All these new ventures were established as Departments providing a clinical service. They broadened the type of patient sent by special referral to Hammersmith, and confirmed what everyone already knew: Hammersmith Hospital received rare and exceptional patients, not the routine patient and his common disease. To some extent this development was inevitable; to a major extent it was encouraged by staff working there. The need for better hospital accommodation, however, was now becoming desperate.

There was no progress in the plea to start building the new hospital even though a Chief Planning Officer had been appointed (the same man returned in 1982 with greater expectations!) although planning for redevelopment was at an advanced stage: 'demolition work on the centre site should start later this year (1973) and who knows we may see the foundations of the new hospital actually beginning in 1975'. Some demolition did occur and £2 million was spent in survey fees and the creation of an untidy car park in the centre of the Hospital on which huts were erected to house the Department of Anaesthetics until a new brick building was put up on the site of their previous home, another hut, of which Anaesthetics would have the first floor and the machinery for Nuclear Magnetic Resonance occupy the ground floor, funded by N.H.S. money and on an N.H.S. site, an unusual opportunity for a University and N.H.S. enterprise. The new hospital, which was expected 'to rise like a phoenix from the old boiler house', never materialized, and the development was postponed officially in April 1975. Instead, the old building became the central office for the seven trades unions located on site.

Second, the Government White Paper on the Framework for Government Research and Development (published in 1971, which stemmed from the reports of Sir Frederick Dainton and Lord Rothschild, with their contrasting views) meant that the Medical Research Council had to surrender £5.5 million out of its modest budget of £22.4 million to the Department of Health and Social Security. The effect on the School was likely to be severe if only because the M.R.C. had become the largest single contributor to the Hammersmith research funds. At that time outside monies supported about 42% of the School budget for staff and research activities and it should be remembered that the four academic departments of 1935 had increased to 15 in 1971. Because of the lack of university finance for clinical advances new posts were paid for by the N.H.S., and as a result the School structure had moved away from the '1951 Agreement'; whereas in 1935 the senior staff were almost entirely full-time University employees, by 1975 the proportion had dropped to 60%.

THE 1974 CHARTER

Third, the School reverted to an independent and presumably self-sufficient body within the University of London, a reversion to its 1935 status. On 25 January 1974 the School received a new charter 'reconstituting it as a University Medical School within Greater London'. It revoked the Royal Charter of 10 July 1931 when the School was founded as 'The British Postgraduate Medical School', revoked the supplemental charter of 31 March 1947 when the name of the School was altered to the 'Postgraduate Medical School of London', revoked the further supplemental charter of 11 September 1967 when the title became 'Royal Postgraduate Medical School'. The School was reconstituted as a University Medical School 'by the name and style of the Royal Postgraduate Medical School'. The charter renewed the purpose of the School: 'the objects of the School shall be the teaching and practice of and research into the science and art of medicine and such allied subjects as may be decided upon from time to time by the Council'. It no longer defined the student body as the 1931 charter had, but it set out the School's powers which included 'to provide, maintain, administer and regulate residential accommodation – (i) for the staff of the School for proper consideration; and (ii) for the students of the School, so far as is necessary to enable them to pursue their studies'.

The charter also gave power 'by agreement to retain and acquire rights to use the site and buildings of Hammersmith Hospital for the objects of the School', which had not appeared in previous charters. To replace the badge of the Postgraduate Medical Federation by which the School had become known, it was allowed 'to obtain through Our College of Arms a grant of armorial bearings which shall be duly recorded in Our said College'. Professor Emeritus Lord Stamp[103] generously donated money for a suitable crest to be drawn and the motto 'Manus medentum dirigit scientia' (knowledge guides the hand of healers'): the crest included an anvil and hammers (an allusion to Hammersmith as the geographical site), the staff of Aesculapius (for medicine), a crown (to indicate that the School was a Royal Chartered body) and a display of wormwood – *Artemisia absinthium* – (more a bow to mythology than truth) and the scroll beneath.

The Academic Board, which had been constituted by the 1947 charter to replace the School Council of the 1931 charter remained. The new School Council was reconstituted as originally, with appointed, elected, and ex-officio members and the power to co-opt. The School could now confer the title of visiting Professor and 'Institute Fellowships, Studentships, Scholarships, Exhibitions, Bursaries, Prizes and other aids to research'. There were many who expected the new charter and new independence within the University to bring freedom from financial restrictions and a larger budget. They were quickly disillusioned and disappointed.

Fourth, there was an unusually large number of retirements of people who had been around when the School was founded – and by implication carried some of the original philosophy and aspirations – and the loss of such staff changed the outlook of newcomers. The Foundation Professors had not surrounded themselves with fawning inferiors – a philosophy as common in medicine and commerce then as it remains today in spite of the obvious long-term disadvantages – but had chosen the best: men who excelled in their own field and who would have been outstanding in any other field whatever the criteria. These people took over the running of a department when the chief was away or retired: most moved away to establish their own units and those who remained became heads in their turn, to continue the tradition of excellence. The Academic Board in 1955 was only 11 people (just double what it had been 20 years earlier); in 1975 there were 36 people (by 1980 there were 43) and already so unwieldy for the running of the School that an 'inner cabinet' (better known as a 'kitchen cabinet' and comparable to the Wilson Government cabinet of 1964) had already begun to evolve.

Much of the decision-making at Hammersmith was elitist, in the sense that elitism permits the domination of decision-making by a single group and with limited access to this process by the rank and file. Most of the rank and file were not interested in detail or in taking part, provided that it remained clear that decisions were being made for the common good. Pareto defined the elite as the best in any field and such people are thus the best to rule: the Hammersmith agreed. Besides, the ruling elite were a well-defined group, certainly from the earliest days, and it was not until the mid-seventies that key decisions ran counter to those of the majority with a resulting unrest, not just among doctors, but throughout the School. With the increase in size of the School there was a loss of easy communication and sense of purpose.

There were similarities between scientific method (as practised by all researchers) and decision-making, which was another reason why decisions were largely left to a small caucus. Unfortunately, decisions are not actually made in a rational way, because rationality requires a complete knowledge and anticipation of the consequence that will follow from each choice but, since the consequences lie in the future, rationality requires a choice among all possible alternatives. In practice, choice is directed by the stimulus, and the stimulus at Hammersmith was 'space'. There was no clearly defined single objective in the 'new school' but a general impetus to turn space into laboratories. Everyone had goals and aspirations and they usually conflicted. Hammersmith did what many organizations still do: attend to one goal at a time and when the first goal has been achieved move on to the next; in this way any conflict between goals is ignored. But the result can be an inexplicable mess to the next generation.

The School had been founded to teach medicine to King George's British Empire, and when that was given away after the war there was nothing to replace it. The British Empire was dissolved in a fairly amiable way, without any disastrous wars to preserve it, which showed that Englishmen realized that the weight of numbers made it impossible to continue with the old system. The loss of the Empire was to some extent a loss of purpose too, but the effects of it were hard to gauge. Perhaps the British Empire was more apparent to foreigners than to the British themselves. To the Hammersmith it did not mean a reduction in student numbers nor loss of recognition abroad; indeed Hammersmith had always been better acknowledged by its peers outside the country than within, probably because its achievements were less well known in the U.K. than they should have been. Empires had fallen before. Britain had not been defeated: she had voluntarily given her Empire away and retired to a small island democracy, an astonishing achievement by any standards. Such a thing had never happened before: there was no bloodshed or chaos in Britain at the loss of Imperial Power, and indeed the withdrawal was made so amicably that a Comonwealth of Nations maintaining a relationship (and in the case of the Hammersmith a very important relationship) of friendship replaced what conquest had acquired in the previous 200 years. What was the Hammersmith to do?

EUROPEAN MEDICINE

The politicians could not make up their minds about Europe: Heath had taken Britain into the Community in 1973, the 1975 referendum was a two-to-one vote in favour of Britain remaining in Community membership although less than 65% of the electorate voted, and even in 1978 there was no evidence that Britain was welcomed in the Common Market. Yet Hammersmith's short specialist courses (started by the Department of Medicine in 1968 and by Surgery the next year) had increasingly attracted attenders from Scandinavia and Western Europe: in the late seventies as many as 65% for some subjects and a demand for more (17 specialist short courses had a total of 1254 attenders in 1977). Hammersmith was, of course much closer to the U.S.A. than Europe – in language, philosophy, training and democratic organization – but the opportunity to play a part in European postgraduate medical education was inviting. America was still the country where more seemed possible than anywhere else; opportunity still beckoned; freedom was still not only pronounced but enforced. Moreover, for the past 10 years the U.K. had been the main participant in the Exchange Professorships between the Medical School of the University of California, Los Angeles, and teaching hospitals in this country. Hammersmith had done well, sending its own and greeting theirs, and liked to think that both benefited. A European link without Government approval might be embarrassing even though many of those attending the Hammersmith courses were americanophile, but with a strong Community spirit.

There was some good news. The *conversazione* on 11 November 1973 was a stately occasion for 500 guests to view just 16 exhibits, a select 5% of what could have been shown, but all at the advancing edges of medicine: the cell in disease, diagnosis by non-invasive techniques and advances in drug treatment. The Du Cane Housing association, for so long just a plan and a promise, materialized when 112 units of accommodation were handed over in 1976. On 11 March of that year H.R.H. Prince Philip K.G., K.T., the Duke of Edinburgh, who had become President of the School in 1975 (the first President had been Field Marshal Lord Alexander of Tunis who died in 1969), visited the School informally. He met staff, saw work in progress, had tea and talked with students; Hammersmith had always appreciated informal visits by Royalty – H.R.H. Princess Anne's visit in 1983 as Chancellor of the University was equally appreciated – not just for the honour paid and the boost to morale but because on those occasions the visitors were knowledgeable and interested in what the School was doing for British Medicine.

There was also Chandigarh, an honourable failure. When India and Pakistan had partitioned the Punjab in 1947, the world-renowned architect, Le Corbusier, was asked to design a city for 100,000 people and a new capital for the eastern part of the state. Chandigarh became the new capital of both the Punjab and Haryana States, as Union Territory in 1966 and in the same year the School was asked to collaborate in developing a postgraduate medical school on the Hammersmith lines. During the first 5 years 17 members of the School staff worked at Chandigarh, usually for 1 year. There was an exchange of staff, export of some very expensive equipment (financed by the Overseas Development Corporation), high-level inspections, and some joint research done. By 1972 the whole development was becoming bogged down in bureaucracy, an evident failure and clearly too ambitious. Two years later the joint enterprise was wound up and quietly abandoned.

The year the quinquennium was stopped Selwyn Taylor resigned as Dean, there was a nurses' strike and a 30% pay award in response, the Industrial Relations Act was repealed, two General Elections were held and Malcolm Godfrey took over the deanship: the incumbent at the Hammersmith had changed but the problem remained the same – how to match money and discovery in medicine.

15

The Crisis Years (1978–1982)

Across the country there was a feeling of confusion and frustration: 1973–1979 was the worst period of inflation in British history and threatened every aspect of national culture. For Hammersmith these were critical years but their full effects were yet to come: there were some who did not believe there was a problem; others could not believe there was a solution; the majority just waited. Recurrent strikes and industrial unrest had occurred throughout the decade culminating in the dispute and large demonstration at the Grunwick film processing centre in December 1977. Although the strike by hospital engineers and supervisors for pay and parity ended late in October 1978, the 'Winter of discontent' was just beginning. Hammersmith Hospital, perhaps more than any other London hospital, suffered frequent and unpredictable stoppages of work which inconvenienced everyone and satisfied none: it was estimated that a strike in one area or another on the 14-acre site occurred, on average, every 12 days. No-one seemed to know what to do to prevent further disruption: doctors tended to accept practices which would not inflame trade unions to cause more inconvenience, but non-medical staff, particularly those with many years of service to School and Hospital, were unhappy. The deadlock was broken at local level by a joint meeting of shop stewards (of five out of the six different unions represented on site) and a small group of senior staff to plan for peace. As a result there was not a single serious stoppage during the next 12 months even though other hospitals in London still suffered.

On 14 February 1979 a 'concordat' was signed between the Government and trades unions which deluded no-one. To add to the misery there were serious blizzards in Britain for which Denis Howell was made Minister for

Snow! In March devolution for Scotland failed to obtain the necessary 49% vote for the proposition and in Wales devolution was rejected overwhelmingly: both had appeared to be important and pressing issues at the time of the 1974 general election. On 3 May 1979 a general election was held again: Margaret Thatcher became the country's first woman Prime Minister and the Conservative Party had an overall majority of 43 seats. The recurring financial crises were not immediately stopped: value-added tax was increased to 15% from 8% and inflation steadily rose again to reach 20%. Hospitals were hard hit. Cuts in expenditure could only be made by reducing staff and closing wards: Hammersmith Hospital did both, but the School too was under pressure and rapidly reaching bankruptcy. Country-wide cuts in hospital expenditure were resisted, notably by the members of the Lambeth, Southwark and Lewisham Area Health Authority in August, who refused to implement them. The Government stripped the A.H.A. of power and put in Commissioners to run the Authority; it was not until 25 February 1980 that the High Court ruled that the Secretary of State had acted outside his legal powers by suspending members of the Authority. Next day the Flowers Report on medical education in London was published, and once more there were to be changes in the medical schools.

UNIVERSITY GRANT CUTS

The Conservative Government had fought the 1979 election on two main promises: to reduce inflation and to reduce personal taxation. The high level of inflation was blamed on the world recession in trade, high pay increases and high public expenditure. The White Paper on proposed cuts in public expenditure was published on 1 November 1979. The message for the Hammersmith was clear: the Government would decide what the level of inflation should be for next year, that sum would be added to this year's grant and any difference would have to be found from within the Hospital or School budgets. The task of containment seemed impossible. Salary and wage increases were still to be awarded nationally above the current level of inflation: for instance in July 1979 doctors and dentists were given a 26% pay rise (and in May 1980 a further 30%) and ancillary workers were obtaining comparable increases. Since both Hospital and School spent 70% of their budgets on salaries and wages the only solution was to reduce staff.

A committee to examine the needs of higher education had been set up by Harold Macmillan in December 1960 under the chairmanship of Lord Robbins, a Professor of Economics, and reported in 1963.[104] The recommendations were accepted in March 1964: expansion of university places to 218,000 over 10 years (double the current number) and expanding higher education as a whole to 390,000 places – based on evidence from the U.S.A., France, West Germany, the Soviet Union, and an opinion that more Britons could benefit from higher education in a modern world (shades of the Haldane Report of 1918) – particularly in technology, applied science, and management. Robbins also wanted to improve the conditions of university staff, not just pay which had declined since the war but also prospects of promotion, accommodation and facilities generally. He wanted a Minister of Arts and Sciences – a recommendation not accepted by the government, but one which Hammersmith regarded with mixed feelings. Encouraged by Lord Hailsham, then Minister of Education, eight new universities were founded. At the same time London University expanded from 16,000 students in all faculties in 1961 to 46,000 in 1981, a larger increase in numbers than the enrolment of all the new universities put together! The University Grants Committee (U.G.C.) acted as a buffer state between the Government which provided the money and the universities which spent it; this arrangement pleased only the academics. No-one asked what the university expansion was for: was it for the pursuit of truth and knowledge as an end in itself or an investment for the future in the new industrial technology for the benefit of the nation? As unemployment began to affect graduates in the late seventies, University education, of the rather poor standard that rapid expansion had dictated, lost its glamour as a means of job certainty.

When Mrs Thatcher became Prime Minister in 1979 the U.G.C. budget was clearly one to be cut. The committee appointed by the then Minister of Education, Mark Carlisle, used two yardsticks by which to measure achievement (and therefore 'value for money'): the value of research grants that universities received, and the number of A-levels of their new students. This system favoured Oxford and Cambridge, reduced London a little, but devastated universities with a large social science element, such as Keele and Essex, as well as some of the smaller mixed universities which had not suffered much unemployment among their graduates (Aston, Salford, and Glasgow for instance). The U.G.C. was made the scapegoat for the cuts in finance and contraction in size of so many universities. Lord Robbins, the exponent of earlier expansion, had since become Chancellor to the new University of Stirling which suffered an 18% cut in the process, and he was not pleased. The polytechnics, which had spawned new buildings with the same ease as the universities, were heavily pruned too. Politicians of all parties had become disillusioned by the promise of a 'white hot technological revolution'.

At the Hammersmith the outlook was grave although few gave much thought to what the outcome might be. Most were too busy pursuing their own research, treating their own patients, teaching their own students – for the Hammersmith was becoming a federation of specialist departments – to worry about events outside. The crisis came in 1980. There had been warnings in the previous 3 years but financial alarms in the past had been resolved so frequently at the last moment that further warnings could not be taken seriously: the Good Fairy would always wave her magic wand, and anyway who would dare to close down such a famous hospital as the Hammersmith?

The true answers were simply not believed by the majority. Yet in the Spring of 1980 there was a minority who believed that neither the Hospital nor the School could survive. The Hospital had never fitted neatly into the classification of teaching and non-teaching hospitals (where teaching meant medical students, and the product was a qualified doctor) ever since the N.H.S. began 30 years earlier; the cost of treating patients was higher than in other hospitals and the buildings were now old and shabby. Clearly there had to be closure of some hospitals 'excess to requirements' because the population in London had fallen, and 2 miles away there was the new, modern Charing Cross Hospital with spare capacity to look after the indigenous population living around the Hammersmith.

FINANCIAL DISASTER

The School depended largely on the University for its money in spite of attempts to increase its income from other sources, and the University was not inclined to increase its allocation even though further savings locally seemed impossible. The Dean held a public meeting of all staff to try to explain that negotations were taking place, but he could not provide details. The impending financial crisis was debated at the Academic Board on several occasions but without a consensus for action. The idea of deliberately overspending was turned down, not so much because Commissioners would be installed to make those cuts that the Academic Board could not bring itself to introduce, but that cuts would be such that any future recovery might become impossible. Others wished to raid the endowment and research funds, although these were in fact too small to salvage the School for more than 6 months: in 1966 these funds had been held centrally and the total had been removed to pay for a financial short-fall at the time: the sum was only £15,000 but had taken many years to accrue, and because of the 'raid' decentralization was demanded and obtained. In 1980, such was the panic that only one voice was raised against the use in an emergency of the R&D funds to pay for salaries, but the voice was enough to obtain the promise of a review of all income.

In fact, the School finances had been slipping out of control for many reasons, the most important being the expansion of work in departments and the creation of new units as medical research develop at an increasing pace. Since 1974 these increased liabilities had been restrained by 'freezing' all but essential vacant staff posts, by reducing the level of departmental running costs, by curtailing the cost of maintenance and repair of premises, and by actively seeking larger grants from charitable bodies. The new crisis was due to three causes.

First, students. The School had never defined the term, but from earliest days it was used to separate permanent staff from travellers. As such, all junior hospital staff were classified as students: when the N.H.S. arrived and junior staff were paid by the State there was no attempt to make a distinction between overseas visitors and hospital juniors. In any case, the fees charged to students were low, almost token, and the number of junior staff relatively small in relation to the total student body. In the 1960s the University attempted to simplify the procedure of payment: a student was someone who stayed for 1 month; the fees paid to the School and thence to the University would in future be deducted in advance from the School's U.G.C. annual allocation, any adjustment being made the following year. With high inflation in the seventies, tuition fees had fallen in value and the School was in effect subsidizing students. Moreover, when the type of teaching changed to the more popular and more convenient 5-day seminar, the number of 'students' declined by definition but the budget was no longer so adjusted.

The U.G.C. recurrent grant for 1978 was £2.415 million, leaving a deficit of £147,000. In 1979 the recurrent grant was £3.162 million and with increased tuition fees provided a surplus of £64,000. In 1980 the Government's new policy on fees for overseas student became effective. The aim was to transfer the direct costs of educating overseas students from the U.G.C. recurrent grant to the individual student who was to be charged an 'economic fee', and the potential total was to be deducted from the School's recurrent grant over a 3-year period. This policy applied to all universities and medical schools, but the School differed notably from others in that by its Charter of 1931 it had an obligation to teach and train overseas students. In 1980 half the School's students came from abroad, compared with the national average of only 13%. Consequently the School stood to lose approximately half of its recurrent grant over the 3-year period 1980–1983, an amount much greater than the sum that could be recovered by tuition fees. The Government subsequently set the maximum fee for a student at £10,000 a year: if the School had settled for this sum the total fee income was, on market research, likely to fall drastically: the School settled for £7000 a year, which was nearly five times the previous annual rate. The government had set up a special fund, to help institutions undertaking postgraduate work of national importance to adjust to the new fees policy, and the School received a grant of £600,000 to add to its annual recurrent grant which had now dropped to £2.726 million. In addition a single grant of £260,000 was received from the University of London Reserves, thus allowing the School to show a surplus of £67,000. The projected budget for 1981/1982 was expected to disclose a deficit of £550,000 by 31 July 1982 with no possibility of further savings or grants. In effect this meant that the School was bankrupt.

THE DAINTON INVESTIGATION AND REPORT

In the light of the report from The Finance and General Purposes Committee of the School Council, the Academic Board approved, on 3 November 1981, the setting up of a Joint Committee on Staffing 'to consider the future structure and staffing of the School and to make recommendations'. The Chairman was Sir Frederick Dainton F.R.S.[105] (who was also Chairman of Council): Mr H. H. Blandford[106] (Treasurer to the School) and Sir Frank Hartley[107] (Chairman of Council Personnel Committee) were both appointed by the School Council and the Academic Board appointed Professor R. B. Welbourn[108] (Chairman of the Academic Board), Professor R. E. Steiner[109] and Professor N. A. Wright[110] from its own members.

This small committee of six people moved fast. It collected evidence from January to March, analysed and discussed the findings with heads of departments in April and presented its 60-page report and recommendations on 20 May 1982. It was the first complete investigation of the activities of the Royal Postgraduate Medical School ever undertaken in its 47 years existence. The results were far-reaching, radical, and provided a reasoned plan for the future. Indeed, when the University Grants Committee issued in 1984, its consultation document 'Higher Education into the 1990's', Hammersmith had almost completely redesigned its organization and was able to respond with authority. The Committee regarded each member of the academic staff as one unit: by questionnaire a profile was provided from the following information:

- Factual details about the staff member such as age, length of service, grade, salary.
- Academic details such as the number of annual publications in the previous 5 years, students attached or working alongside for a thesis.
- Involvement in short courses in the past 5 years and the income from tuition fees.
- General duties undertaken for the School.
- Type and amount of clinical work undertaken (where appropriate), details of support from N.H.S. staff, and reimbursement monies by the N.H.S. for services provided by the School, including private fees 'income'.
- Research grants held in the previous 4 years and their value.
- Details of staff supported on 'soft money' where such grants depended on the work of the member of the academic staff.
- Details of 'hard money' supported staff dependent on the work of the member of the academic staff.

Analysis of the questionnaires enabled the costs and benefits to the School to be established and by collating under academic departments, a departmental profile could be created and discussed with the head of the current 13 departments. The cost of teaching was to be measured by tuition fees and the cost of research by the grants attracted, both of which were used in the criteria for identifying posts to be discontinued.

Four senior members of staff agreed to retire early, and two secretaries accepted redundancy, but the savings amounted only to £98,000. The concept of 'across the board' reduction in staffing was rejected in favour of a selective approach which could preserve the essential character and unique value of the institution. It was realized that in industry there are often many workers performing identical tasks, and that the number of staff can be reduced in any group by an agreed percentage: the jobs to be made redundant being selected first by asking for volunteers and then by applying a uniform policy of 'last-in/first-out' dismissal, as had been practised during the previous decade in manufacturing and heavy industries in Britain. The Committee attempted to identify those academic and clinical activities which, if lost, would not destroy the viability of the School to maintain its multi-disciplinary character yet preserve its clinical services for the N.H.S. Hence there was no general call for staff to retire early, and only those volunteers were accepted where the staff member would not need to be replaced.

The task was not easy. Some recommendations meant that members of staff who had given long and distinguished service to the School would be asked to leave. There was also the real danger that the institution would have too many young people and too few of the older and more experienced to guide future developments. The posts identified were to be disestablished on 31 December 1982. The total savings came to nearly £347,000, leaving a considerable shortfall. There was one further complication. As part of the Government's policy to reduce expenditure in the Public Sector 'volume cuts' of 7½% in each of the next 2 years were to be introduced which would raise the School deficit to an annual £600,000 by 1983/1984. The term 'volume cuts' needs explanation: it is a Civil Service term to mean a volume of activity, and a cut meant a reduction in the baseline of a grant, not merely a reduction in the money calculated for inflation: this meant a reduction in size in absolute terms and not just standing still. It was the death blow to the future of the School.

The Dean, Dr Malcolm Godfrey, wrote to the Vice-Chancellor outlining the future financial state of the School and the difficulty of maintaining the '1951 Agreement' by which the University provided consultant services to Hammersmith Hospital. The University was asked to take account of the need to maintain the research base of the School in grant allocations: there was talk of how research of importance within the University might be suitably protected but no judgement on the meaning of 'importance'. In addition, informal discussions took place with the Department of Health and Social Security about the clinical services for the Hospital. It is worth recording that the N.H.S., although the sole employer of doctors and nurses in Britain, had taken little part in education, training, standards nor research since its inception. Article 3 of the School Charter of 1974 had specifically outlined the objects of the School: 'The objects of the School shall be the teaching and practice of and research into the science and art of medicine and such allied subjects as may be decided upon from time to time by Council.' Since 1970, the School had provided 58 Professors (24 for the United Kingdom), 63 Readers and Senior Lecturers (41 for the U.K.) and 90 Lecturers (62 for the U.K.); 56

Hammersmith postgraduates had been appointed to U.K. teaching hospitals and 52 to similar posts abroad. The number of research publications from the School had averaged 500–600 annually. Monies raised for research from grant-giving bodies (such as the Medical Research Council, the Wellcome Trust, Nuffield Foundation and two dozen others) had matched the recurrent grant from the University ever since 1966. In 1980/1981 the recurrent grant was £2.726 million and the School's 'earned' income was £4.597 million. For an institute to provide 63% of its own support is no mean performance, but it would not be possible for the School to be completely self-supporting, however desirable.

It was when one examined staff that some disquieting features emerged. Research at the Hammersmith had been related essentially to care and cure of patients: the results of research were rapidly evaluated and introduced into clinical practice at Hammersmith Hospital, whence they spread through the country and abroad. The oft-quoted complaint that new methods discovered by research were not applied in the N.H.S. was not accepted: medical progress in the past 10 years, for example, argued quite to the contrary. But research results depended on people and grants. The Dainton Report discovered that whereas technical staff were almost equally supported by University and research grant monies (185 and 122 persons), research staff were almost entirely dependent on non-University funds (10 University to 96 non-University). Of the medical staff in 1982, 77 were full-time University (plus 13 full-time on grant monies) and 13 part-time, whereas 156 were full-time N.H.S.: the latter were essentially junior staff, as expected by the '1951 Agreement', but did include 15 Consultants full-time and 14 part-time. This represented a departure from the '1951 Agreement' principle even though such N.H.S. Consultant staff were of high academic quality and played their part in the work of the School. The Dainton Committee appreciated that this agreement meant that clinical practice, teaching and research were inextricably and beneficially (for University and N.H.S.) interwoven – whereas separation would have made their cost-cutting exercise much simpler – and that each component depended upon the other so that changes in one activity had far-reaching implications for the other. Even so, the Committee considered that the '1951 Agreement' should be preserved and restored as far as possible. The Committee disestablished 24 posts, and added these to the 22 post already 'frozen' since 1974.

The Committee wrote: 'There can be no doubt whatsoever that our proposals will damage the School and its ability to provide clinical services . . . we are confident that the School – although smaller in size – will be able to continue to advance postgraduate medical education and research and have a secure base from which to grow again in happier times . . . if the School has to reduce the number of staff still further to meet this deficit (of £600,000 from volume cuts) it would mean the disestablishment of a further 18 academic (consultant) and 18 supporting staff posts. The number of full-time academic staff would then have fallen from 65 at the beginning of the 1981/1982 academic year to 35 by 1984 – a reduction of 46%. The reduction in full-time academic staff over the 10-year period 1974–1984 (taking into account posts frozen in the period 1974–1982) would be from 78 to 35, a reduction of 55%.' The report explored various possibilities, including academic collaboration with St Mary's Hospital Medical School, but these would not have saved any money, and concluded: 'The time-scale for action is exceedingly short and those with the responsibility for academic and health service work in this country must now decide whether or not the Royal Postgraduate Medical School is to continue to play its important part in the development of British Medicine. The necessary solution to preserve the RPMS as a national institution can no longer be found by local decision.'

THE NEW ERA

By the Spring of 1983 the recommended reduction in staff members and in other expenditure had been put into effect without excessive damage to the work of the School. The University of London recognized that, in spite of depleted resources, the maintenance of high-quality research at the School must receive priority, and accepted the School's contention that it represented a centre of excellence in British Medicine. Accordingly, the University increased its recurrent grant for the year so that the School had a sound financial basis on which to build. But friends also came to the aid of the Hammersmith.

First, there were two major benefactions from charitable funds. The Wolfson Foundation agreed to support the work of the Department of Clinical Pharmacology to the extent of £100,000 each year for 5 years, and the British Heart Foundation endowed half a million pounds for the salary and costs of a Professor of Cardiac Surgery. Both of these generous benefactions have helped preserve two established and well-recognized departments.

Second, the Medical Research Council conferred Research Group status, therefore in effect underwriting the cost of research programmes, on the work being directed by Professor Batchelor (immunology), Professor Bloom (endocrinology), Professor Dollery (clinical pharmacology), Professor Luzzatto (haematology), Professor Peters (renal medicine), and Dr Pepys (immunological medicine). The recognition thus gained was particularly welcomed because it represented an endorsement of the research activities of the academic staff of the School after the most rigorous scrutiny by their scientific peers.

Third, the staff of the School continued to solicit grants for research projects as it had done in the past, in competition with other institutions, but with a 23% increase in success.

Fourth, the School set up a Jubilee Appeal to raise funds to further research into the diagnosis and treatment of disease, with the aim of establishing an endowment of £3 million. Two previous appeals had received support from the national and international community who sympathized with the objectives of the Hammersmith and who benefit from the contributions that School and Hospital make to medical knowledge. The first appeal in 1954 conceived the new and larger medical school with ample laboratories, the second in 1968 allowed the expansion and development of work in the new building. This third appeal might cushion the School against any sudden future, painful reductions as had been necessary in 1982.

16

1984 and The Way Ahead

Hammersmith has resisted the inclination to present bland generalizations as acknowledged facts. Even so, those over-anxious in the seventies might be seen as over-confident in the eighties. None of the measures listed in the last chapter will solve the School's problems for more than a few years: they did not mean that the School could relax; rather that breathing space had been given for the School to become financially resilient and insure that the drift into bankruptcy would never be allowed to occur again. The School and Hospital would now be forced to become more aggressive and more efficient, even enterprising, to claim a secure future. The R.P.M.S. had not reached a stage of perfection, nor was it free from danger. Problems and tensions remain. In the lives of institutions there are very seldom clear breaks with the past, but the past few years had forced the School to reform faster and more radically then it would have done.

There is no clear indication that there is a role for the Hammersmith as a centre of excellence or what contribution it should make towards the national provision of medical education. In 1981 it was preoccupied with survival, a spectre that has not wholly disappeared with the recognition of the Hospital as a Special Health Authority. The present Government has created a climate in which independence and excellence are not regarded as anti-social; it has not said that Hammersmith should be kept open at any price. Independent medicine is a service industry: if a private hospital cannot attract customers it will go out of business. In many ways Hammersmith is similar. The aim of those who manage the School's affairs must be to provide an educational service that doctors want to buy, at a cost they can afford. Incompetent management whether of the School's education provision or of its finances will put the School's future at risk, as will the failure to respond effectively to the challenge of change. It may well be that the clientele of the Hammersmith will not decrease as much under the impact of raised fees as expected. New customers are already coming from new lands, but as the 1983 Annual Report made clear some of these doctors lack an adequate understanding of the English language and good basic medical training.

The School must still retain the clear policy of a coherent educational philosophy, which has been so successful for the past 50 years and made the place a unique institution. In 1984 the Royal Postgraduate Medical School, Hammersmith Hospital, and four Medical Research Council Units together form a centre of world-wide fame and reputation for clinical practice and clinical research – 'the Hammersmith'. Undoubtedly the Hammersmith owed its strength and success to its unique organization, established in 1935 during the austerity of 'the Depression', by men of vision who recognized that London needed a true university hospital – led by academics – to promote the development of scientific medicine.

There are probably new sources of revenue that could be developed, or at least could be the subject for properly conducted feasibility studies: the Hammersmith may need to overturn the traditional amateurism and reluctance to exploit the financial possibilities of the School. The key figure in this change will be the School Secretary who should be the permanent head of administration (the Civil Service side) – and the Dean the head of academic organization (the educational side) – which makes him the chief executive of the School: in practice the two cannot be separated or made simple, and must work in harmony.

Most of the new capital raised by previous School appeals (a total of over £4 million) was spent on buildings rather than on scholarships and bursaries: admittedly in other institutions where these are available they are frequently and disappointingly not taken up. The money raised for research, now averaging an annual £5 million and about equal to the University Grant, has been from the efforts and imagination of individual staff, but these efforts have neither been co-ordinated nor directed. From 1970 to 1980 staff members raised the considerable sum of £12 million. The Dainton Committee recommendations of 1982 were based partly on the earning power of individual units: it would be tragic if this were the sole criterion for retaining special units, but clearly it has to be a major consideration in policy. The excellence of patient care must be a key qualification for preserving the link between Hospital and School. One without the other would not survive, nor would there be a reason to attempt to save either. The School has always dominated the Hospital, which was to be expected, and this had been accepted from the earliest days: the London County Council doctors appointed to the four foundation professorial units were in name only.

Drucker[111] often insisted that every enterprise should ask and answer two questions: What business are we in? What do we do best? He believed that business enterprises and public-service institutions (and Hammersmith is a bit of both) are organs of society. They do not exist for their own sake but to fulfil a specific social purpose and to satisfy a specific need of society. 'They are not ends in themselves but means. The right question to ask in respect of them is not, What are they? but, What are they supposed to be doing and what are their tasks?' So what is Hammersmith supposed to be doing and what is its task in 1984? It continues to treat patients and teach students, and both are still founded on research. Yet there have been changes – some subtle, some marked. In clinical practice the institution has become a tertiary referral centre – for patients treated by specialists in their own fields who wish another opinion or further expertise – but remains essentially a diagnostic mecca. Hence the greater proportion of patients admitted to some units has become the rare, the unusual, the incredible and the unbelievable, with the inevitable criticism of inspectors of higher training of the Royal Colleges. There appears to be no easy solution. Hammersmith needs jobs approved for higher training (which will lead to accreditation in any particular subject, and hence the ability of its students to apply for consultant posts) yet cannot really afford to compromise in the type of patient or condition being managed. The N.H.S. is unhelpful, the Royal Colleges are inflexible.

FUTURE PROSPECTS

No-one in his right mind would attempt to predict the future of Hammersmith. No historian could: as a matter of discipline he is trained to look backwards, to interpret, to analyse and to synthesize as best he can. But the temptation to look ahead is irresistible. Prediction is a dangerous enterprise: at various times people have predicted that the wireless would kill the gramophone, that television would ruin radio, that further medical advances would not come. All were wrong and for a variety of reasons, the commonest being that the evidence of change was there but not looked for.

For the historian of political and social events of this century, the main divisions seem inevitable: the beginning of the Great War in 1914, the Great Depression of 1929–1932, the end of the Second World War in 1945, and the Recovery of the 1980s are the decisive punctuation marks. They were the important dates in world history for Britain. Historians may well decide that the five pivotal dates for the Hammersmith were 1916, 1935, 1951, 1974 and 1981. In 1916 Hammersmith became a special Hospital, an experimental hospital although the nature of the experiment was not appreciated at the time. In 1935 postgraduate education in medicine was organized on the basis of a general hospital and probably on the right lines. In 1951 agreement was reached on the position of full-time University academics in the N.H.S., but the price was high: the Hammersmith had been weakened by the competition of the market place because although private practice may not destroy the ethos, failure to respond to drift may be more damaging. In 1974 Hammersmith reverted to being an independent School in the University, thus ending an unproductive sacrifice, and in 1982 it became a Special Health Authority within a reorganized health service. A reorganized N.H.S., and particularly an S.H.A., should do what Christopher Hogg[112] did for Courtaulds and Lord Weinstock[113] for General Electric (and there are many other examples of imaginative enterpreneurs): both were ailing companies in the seventies. Both men set targets and cash limits for their companies and then left them alone: both companies responded and did well. The N.H.S. has suffered from a surfeit of well-meant advice in the past but this is no longer required nor welcomed.

There are four areas which should be explored: private practice and the salaries of staff, the funding and direction of research, organization and performance, and finally buildings.

PRIVATE PRACTICE

The Goodenough Report of 1944 (p. 17, para. 8) stated: 'On the question of whether whole-time clinical professors should be allowed a limited amount of private practice, and if so, on what terms, it is felt that the vital matter is to appoint as professors, persons of the right outlook. If this is to be done, whatever rule is made regarding the professor's contacts with private patients will be of minor importance. But the professor should be protected from pressure to see patients other than in exceptional circumstances. It is thought that generally the most satisfactory form of protection will be secured by allowing the professor the right to attend a limited number of private patients, normally on the premises of the teaching hospital, but to stipulate that he shall not receive any fees from them.' This was no solution, just deferment of two questions that many were to ask and no-one to answer: first, should Professors be allowed to augment their income by private practice for any reasons at all and second, will their performance as researchers and teachers be harmed thereby? In 40 years no private practice has been allowed in the University of London in the faculty of Medicine but has been allowed in Law, Engineering and most other faculties – a curious anomaly that persists. Other Universities, notably Manchester and Oxford, have allowed Professors to practise medicine for personal gain and have attempted to regulate these gains, with certain restrictive university obligations: many universities in the U.S.A. have compromised similarly on this issue. Forty years after Goodenough an acceptable solution seems no nearer, yet the matter is urgent: there was evidence in 1982 that academic posts were not being filled because of their poor financial prospects, a situation likely to worsen.

McMichael frequently stated that young people wishing to devote a career to academic medicine should expect to be paid less than full-time clinicians: their reward lay in the discovery of new knowledge – but new knowledge can be put to good use for the patients' benefit by the full-time clinician and for his material benefit. The argument is tenuous. Besides, there is a limit to the level of sacrifice. The *Association of University Teachers Bulletin* (in 1977) published some interesting comparisons of incomes: the income of working-class wages went up more between 1938 and 1976 than the salaries of many professional people: for the factory worker the increase was 172% of the purchasing power of the 1938 wage, for the coal-miner 256%, agricultural worker 199%, bus-driver 144%, solicitor 98%, graduate school-teacher 95%, general medical practitioner 81% and university professor 74%. In medicine the merit-award scheme has gone some way to improve incomes, but even in 1983 many Professors were known not to be in receipt of any award: the 'A' award added about 50% to the pre-taxed salary but the 'C' award was little more than a generous 'pour-boire'. Yet a surgeon in private practice had only to operate on one patient a week to double his N.H.S. salary, and many were earning five times the top academic salaries in 1982. In the past 3 years, as private practice and independent private hospitals have become better organized, the differentials have increased.

There is a piece of doctrine, which sees a conflict of interest between public good and private profit. There has never been any firm evidence for this. What has to be admitted is that the time available for research and private practice is limited. Time used on one must inevitably be subtracted from the other. Few people seem to realize just how difficult it is to generate original thought, on how time-consuming its development into a practical project can be. By comparison, the application of the acquired and special skills of a good doctor are cheaper in time and effort – and with a measurable and easily recognizable result – than creative thought which may produce no result. When the two are in competition, the thought processes become financial sacrifices.

The term 'academic' is currently used as a word of abuse. This is sloppy and incorrect. Academic means 'of belonging to a learned society' in its broadest sense, according to the dictionary, an excellent characteristic of man and certainly preferable to ignorance. Even McMichael admitted in 1980 (12 years after retirement) that staff at the Hammersmith possessed skills which were undervalued and could command much money in the open market. The dilemma persists, but will have to be faced boldly and solved wisely, and soon. Certainly in 1984 the arguments for limited private practice for university staff seem irrefutable, the debate being about control not denial. Experience in the U.S.A. indicates that everyone benefits and that the disadvantages have been over-emphasized, sometimes maliciously so.

DIRECTION OF RESEARCH

There will always be a need for research in medicine and a shortage of funds and facilities. It is appropriate that attempts should be made to establish priorities so that research is directed to specific problems and questions in the provision of services to patients and populations. Hammersmith has so far largely pursued individual initiatives, and successfully so, but one question neglected today is the relationship between research and the need to change services – commonly called 'operational research'.

Kearns in 1984[114] commented that the National Health Service uses the word 'research' differently from other organizations, possibly because of the emphasis the medical profession places on it, as a matter for individual initiative and for special funding rather than being seen as an essential function of management: 'It is a curiosity that many social services departments have research officers on their establishments while most health authorities do not'. Few at the Hammersmith would agree to delegate research, yet most would have to concede that there are neglected areas. Industrial and commercial organizations use the phrase 'research and development' to mean something rather different from what the Hammersmith has been doing for the past 50 years.

The study of how we do things, in the modern idiom 'performance indicators', has had little appeal to staff, but is likely to loom large in the future. Hammersmith has done little operational research: only two ventures are noteworthy. The first was the realization and practical demonstration that at least 25% of all surgery (50% of plastic surgery at Hammersmith and the West Middlesex Hospitals, a figure maintained for 2 years) could be done as day cases, without the need of patients to enter hospital and involve the admissions procedure (and thus save substantial overheads, including the cost of a bed). An internal report in 1978 described the management, discipline, variety and results of treating 10,000 patients in 10 years without mishap.[115] The second was the D.I.Y. centre of medical illustration already referred to in the section on photography. The need for this kind of research is desperate for the survival of the N.H.S. in its present form. Hammersmith is well placed (by techniques, knowledge and expertise) to tackle many of the current problems; whether staff will do so is quite a different matter. Yet the questions to be asked and answered are of national and international interest. Unfortunately Health Services Research, the current term for operational research, does not have the scientific basis that Hammersmith uses in diseases research: to measure blood-pressure is one thing, to measure attitudes and behaviour quite another. It may be that grants for this kind of research are hard to come by when compared with the £4.9 million staff raised in 1983 for 'disease oriented' projects. But in 1972 the School did set up a Research Advisory Committee to 'co-ordinate endeavours on this site while at the same time protecting the right of the individual to pursue research as he would wish'. It was an impossible dream and the committee died.

ORGANISATION

There will be much talk of organisation, structures, aims, and management in the future: the NHS had started on all these in 1983 by the Rayner[116] scrutinies for savings and the Griffiths Report on the need for general managers at Regional, District, and Unit levels. The aims of the School have been clear from the start, and this book tries to describe them and record their achievement. Curiously, it is politicians who press for changes in the NHS, yet Britain as a Country is run by permanent civil servants (who ensure continuity of management, but accept modifications dictated by political party doctrines) rather than by politicians. 'Management is not like a career, it's like the church, a calling. You have to have enormous faith and enormous belief in the need to make your enterprise successful'[117]. The Hammersmith has traditionally taken the line that organisation follows aims and people: the most sophisticated management structure in the world will produce poor results if it is filled with second-rate people. Find first-class people and they will quickly find what is the best structure and lead into it without fuss. Hammersmith has been picking outstanding people for 50 years (and so have many successful commercial enterprises). The N.H.S. has been plagued with nostrums for improving its management: Hammersmith largely ignored them. Research clinicians who regularly raise large sums of money must have certain inherent management abilities, and any organization which attempts to provide the public with its single most important source of medical postgraduate education must be run by men and women who are able and sensitive and who, above all, have integrity. The job of the Hammersmith was to make sure that there was an adequate supply of people so qualified: that nearly all seemed to go to the Commonwealth was not really the fault of the staff because (as with the D.C.P. Course, which was the best in the land) the candidates came mainly from overseas and few of our own benefited. Management structures were considered almost irrelevant: they were there for guidance when things went wrong, when individuals drifted away from the general purpose of the School, or there were problems created by personality clashes of which Hammersmith had its full share.

BUILDINGS

Hammersmith has always had a strange addiction for hutted accommodation. In 1950 more exciting research went on in huts than in the brick buildings of the School, and any entrepreneur with about £1000 could purchase premises and site his accommodation wherever space was available; the fact that a hut was placed on any old flat roof and that power was taken from the nearest supply rarely bothered others. At various times the units for the study of Chronic Bronchitis, Cardiopulmonary Blood Flow, Anaesthetics, Paediatrics and several other developing subjects were so housed. Hence the photograph representation of the new hospital-to-be which appeared in the Annual Report by the Board of Governors for Hammersmith Hospital of 1972, showing pitched roofs, was clearly spurious. Flat roofs are still mandatory for any new building: huts may be eyesores but they are convenient, cheap and effective.

The workhouse-hospital designed by a mediocre architect in conventional late Victorian style at the beginning of the Edwardian era and constructed by a competent builder has withstood 80 years of use and alterations. Recent hospital building is another matter. The majority of new buildings since 1960 have been steel-cladded brick buildings, commonplace in any industrial estate, but ugly and unworthy to complement the well-known front entrance.

By contrast, the School had commissioned new buildings in the modern material of cast concrete and then added floors after construction had started as though such action didn't matter. Two have been in trouble. The M.R.C. Cyclotron building of four floors completed in 1954, but extended to eight floors and reopened in 1959, was having expensive new foundations injected in 1984, having had end-supports fitted in 1976. The Commonwealth Building of 10 floors and two basements, originally an eight-storey design, required expensive surface-sealing of its high-alumina concrete in 1983: this had the effect of making the building look cleaner and has to some extent filled in the rough surface of the 'sawn-wood' finish of the original castings that were previously (and unevenly) filled with soot. Neither building compares aesthetically with the red brick of the hospital.

Finally, whatever the outcome of the Hammersmith in the future there is little doubt that those who worked there sought to understand medicine and in seeking found great satisfaction, and as Socrates said more than 2000 years ago, 'there is nothing to match the satisfaction of understanding'. In this respect, the Hammersmith has unfinished business and the ability to carry on, and seems prepared to continue to live dangerously.

17

Annotated References and Notes

My story is of the great equivocation between what was said and what was done, what was promised and what was intended; it also says something, and not a negligible something, about the limits of the influence of that equivocation. It says that there are ways of making better doctors.

Readers who are historians may object that mine is no proper kind of history, neither fish nor fowl, and the objection would be reasonable. Yet the Royal Postgraduate Medical School, as a corporate body, in some of its leading features and in many of its phases was that kind of anomalous and unsatisfactory creature: some insight into its elusive and ambiguous emotions will be useful for anyone attempting to discover the truth. These are the truths, in so far as I have known and understood them, that I wished to convey. I have tried to tell it simply as it was.

As far as the sources of this truth are concerned they are chiefly in oral testimony and personal observation, but also in some official records. The Annual Reports of the School, from 1936 until the present day, and those of Hammersmith Hospital 1952–1974 have been invaluable sources, Others follow in these notes.

CHAPTER 2

1. Addison was extremely able and has been rather neglected by medical historians. Originally a Liberal M.P. he joined the Labour Party in 1929 and became M.P. for Swindon, Wilts. He was a personal friend and adviser to Clement Attlee, Prime Minister in the 1945 Labour Government. He was much in favour of the N.H.S.: perhaps because of him the negotiations between the Minister, Aneurin Bevan, and the Specialists were cordial in contrast to those with the General Practitioners which were not. He was made a Viscount in 1945 and was Chairman of the Medical Research Council in 1948. Addison was author of several books on politics and with Major J. W. Jennings the 12th edition of Ellis's *Demonstrations in Anatomy*. He died in 1951 aged 82.
2. Mackenzie, W. J. M. (1979) *Power and Responsibility in Health Care: the National Health Service as a political institution*, Oxford University Press for the Nuffield Provincial Hospitals Trust, London. Mackenzie was Professor of Politics at Glasgow University 1966–1974, now Emeritus. His account is very readable and pertinent today.

3. Lord Athlone, later to become Chancellor of the University of London (which became centralized by the building of the Senate House in 1929) was Chairman of the Committee which first met in January 1921 and reported 4 months later (*Report of the Post-graduate Medical Committee*, 31 May 1921, HMSO, London). It was very speedy but the recommendations were on an imperial scale.
4. Sir Jonathan Hutchinson died in June 1913 aged 85, having been knighted when he was 80. His son was also consultant surgeon at the London Hospital and died in 1933 aged 74.
5. Newman, C. E. (1966) 'A brief history of the Postgraduate Medical School', *Postgrad. Med. J.*, **42**, 738–740. He was also the author of an unsigned booklet published to mark the Golden Jubilee of the Hospital – *Hammersmith Hospital and the Postgraduate Medical School.* Charles Newman was a governor of St Clement Danes School next door, 1955–1976, and Harveian Librarian at the Royal College of Physicians 1962–1979.
6. *Report of the Postgraduate Education Committee*, April 1930 (set up in July 1925). HMSO, London.
7. The 12 Teaching General Hospitals in London at that time had a total of 5301 beds and 3264 medical students.
8. In 1930 the L.C.C. took over a variety of hospitals – acute services, chronic diseases, fever hospitals, sanatoria, infirmaries: the L.C.C. acquired 29 general hospitals and 18,074 beds. Professor C. L. Mowat (1955, *Britain between the Wars*, Methuen, London) stated that there were 3029 hospitals in Britain of which 1013 were voluntary but only 116 general hospitals) and 523 were Poor Law Hospitals.
9. Viscount Chelmsford (1868–1933) had been Viceroy of India 1916–1921, a Barrister and Warden of All Souls College, Oxford.
10. Sir William Goodenough was on the Governing Body of the School 1937–1943 and then chaired the inquiry into the future of postgraduate institutes in London: *Report of Inter-departmental Committee on Medical Schools*, 1944. HMSO, London.

CHAPTER 3

11. It was said that Walter Long was 'an excellent example of the country squire in politics'. He was created Viscount in 1921 and made First Lord of the Admiralty 1918–1921.
12. The White City Stadium was erected in 1906 for the Olympic Games of 1908 and also used for the Anglo-French Exhibition.
13. The Medical Superintendent was in complete charge of the hospital: many were autocratic. The Goodenough Committee deliberately downgraded the post.
14. For a 400-bed hospital there were, until the Second World War, only four doctors: physician, surgeon, obstetrician, and medical superintendent (who was paid double the salary of the others). Even in 1939 the total cost of the doctors only came to about £2000.
15. See photographs of the old nurses' home and compare with the new: and see Newman, ref. 5.
16. Watson, F. (1934) *Life of Sir Robert Jones*, Hodder & Stoughton, London. Chapter 12 refers to 'Shepherd's Bush'. Jones, a Liverpool graduate, met Dame Agnes Hunt, a nurse with equally progressive ideas, and together they established a Centre for Crippled Children at Baschurch in 1920. Jones was knighted in 1917 and made a Baron in 1920; he died in 1933.

CHAPTER 4

17. Sir Allen Daley – *Hammersmith Hospital* (1951), The Medical Press, 226, 281–285 – wrote of his personal experiences. Lady Daley became the first President of The Friends of Hammersmith Hospital.
18. The duties of the Dean and the correspondence are in the Minute Book of 1933. He was to be paid a salary of £1800; the School Secretary only £421 and the shorthand typist £131.
19. From a note written in longhand on a single sheet of foolscap, undated, in the Archives of the R.P.M.S.

20. McMichael, J. (1966) 'The Postgraduate Medical School: the present situation', *Postgrad. Med. J.*, **42**, 740–743. That bill was paid, but not until 1939.
21. Looking back, MacKeith probably had a raw deal: he was not used to university administration or to adventurous professors.
22. The full-time salary of £2500 was contested, yet Grey Turner in Newcastle, the best-known surgeon outside London, was probably earning £20,000 a year from private practice at the time; coming to Hammersmith was a considerable financial sacrifice.
23. Francis Fraser (1885–1964) was also Director of the British Postgraduate Medical Federation 1945–1960, and Vice-Chancellor of the University 1947–1949.
24. James Young (1883–1963).
25. Edgar Kettle did not want to come to the School, and took a lot of persuading: as a concession to him (more likely than for anyone else) pathology was to be considered as four distinct disciplines and so organized at the School. The others agreed to three at first and to the fourth only in time for the offical opening. Kettle married Marguerite Henrietta on the day she qualified as a doctor in 1918 at St Mary's Hospital where he was the pathologist: she become Assistant Editor to the *Lancet* in 1937 and died in 1939 aged 52. Kettle, probably a sick man when he joined the School, died on 1 December 1936 aged 54, having been made F.R.S. the same year.
26. Grey Turner died in August 1951, aged 73. His son, Elston, became Secretary to the British Medical Association and died in 1983.
27. Chassar Moir (1900–1977) became Nuffield Professor of Obstetrics and Gynaecology in the University of Oxford at the Radcliffe Infirmary for 30 years (1937–1967) and then Visiting Professor at the Hammersmith: he was a familiar face around the place in the seventies.
28. R. S. Aitkin, a New Zealander, was Reader in Medicine 1935–1938 and became Regius Professor of Medicine at Aberdeen 1938–1948, Vice-Chancellor University of Otago 1948–1953 and of Birmingham 1953–1968. He was knighted in 1960 and a member of the University Grants Committee 1968–1973.
29. L. C. Rogers (1897–1961) became Professor of Surgery at the National University of Wales at Cardiff.
30. E. J. King (1901–1962) was Professor of Chemical Pathology from 1944 to 1962, although not a medical man.
31. A. A. Miles became Professor of Bacteriology at University College Hospital in 1937 and Professor of Experimental Pathology 1952–1971. He was knighted in 1966 and became Director of the Lister Institute. (Dr John Gray was made Reader in Morbid Anatomoy in January 1935.)

CHAPTER 5

32. J. H. Laws was at the School 1955–1967 when he became Director and Professor of Radiology at Kings College Hospital.
33. Frank Doyle became Professor of Radiological Science at the School in 1975.
34. Robert Steiner's appointment was probably delayed to save money. He became Professor of Diagnostic Radiology in 1961.
35. The first Cyclotron was built on site by the M.R.C. staff.
36. He came in 1935 and retired in May 1966, a great character.
37. Left in 1940.
38. J. G. Robson was Wellcome Research Professor of Anaesthesia at McGill University, Montreal, before becoming the first Professor of Anaesthesia at the School in 1964. Knighted 1982.
39. McMichael in a recorded interview with Professors Moss and Hill in 1980.
40. Professor Henry Dible died on 1 July 1971.
41. Hitler deliberately bombed the Whitechapel area of London where the working-class Jewish population lived. He used whistling bombs to frighten them: they did. The first air raid was on the evening of the Sabbath and by next day there were 200 corpses laid out in the basement of the London Hospital (mainly blast injuries), thus effectively reducing the

hospital to little more than a casualty-clearing station. The raids continued and medical students could not continue their studies. As one of those, the author found the Hammersmith Local Authority Hospital a rather crummy place and just as noisy because anti-aircraft guns were sited on the Scrubs at the back of the hospital.

42. Thomson, D. (1979) *England in the Twentieth Century: 1914–1963*, Penguin, Harmondsworth.
43. In 1939 many people thought that London would be laid waste overnight but nothing happened except that Poland disappeared. London did endure bombing for 57 consecutive nights in 1940 and for many discontinuous nights until 1944. The multiplier is from Taylor, A. J. P. (1965) *English History 1914–1945*, Clarendon Press, Oxford.
44. West, N. (1981) *M.I.5. Security Service Operations 1909–1945*, The Bodley Head, London.
45. *Hospital Surveys 1945*, HMSO, London.
46. This is also the concern in 1984 as the population shifts south.
47. Written by McMichael in the 1944 Annual Report of the School.

CHAPTER 6

48. Beveridge, W. (1943) *Social Insurances and Allied Services*, HMSO, London. Sir William was an economist and his wife was Secretary and Acting Dean of the London School of Economics and Political Science 1919–1938: she wrote a book, *Beveridge and his Plan*, in 1954 and died in 1959. He was made a Baron in 1946. One observer said of his Report that 'it was uncluttered by evidence': perhaps a bit unfair?
49. Korner, E. (1982) *Steering Group on Health Services Information. First Report to the Secretary of State*, HMSO, London.
50. Goodenough, see ref. 10, and also Pickering, G. W. (1962) *Postgraduate Education and the Specialties with special reference to the Problem in London*, HMSO, London.
51. Lord Robbins, a professor of Economics and later the first Chancellor of Stirling University (1966–1978), had been asked to examine the need for higher education by Harold Macmillan in 1960 and reported to Sir Alec Douglas-Home in March 1964. Dr Jacob Bronowski, Director-General of the National Coal Board's process development department and a well-known writer and broadcaster, had written to *The Times* newspaper (17 September 1963) that unless the status of science and scientists were upgraded quickly, Britain would be 'relegated to the status of a third-class power'. Hence the speed.

CHAPTER 7

52. This applied to most of the countries in Europe which had had enough of the old regimes. *The Times* Weekly Edition of 22 January 1947 had an article about the School under the caption 'School for Doctors'.
53. Ian Aird (1905–1962). When he finally obtained the Surgical Research Laboratories in the Cyclotron Building in 1959, a green marble plaque was placed on the fifth floor entrance, 'Experimental Surgical Unit provided by the Wellcome Trust and the University of London'. In front of this was his own Mynah bird in its cage to greet visitors, often saying 'stop it Heather' (a reference to Aird's daughter and evidence that the bird had spent years at his home: the bird died of old age in 1968).
54. McMichael became Director of the British Postgraduate Medical Federation 1966–1971 and Chris Booth followed him as Professor of Medicine 1966–1977, to be followed by Keith Peters. Booth was made Director of the Clinical Research Centre of the M.R.C. at Northwick Park Hospital in 1978 and knighted 1983.
55. Guillebaud, C. (1956) *Report of the Committee of Enquiry into the Cost of the National Health Service*, HMSO, London.
56. Richard Crossman did raise the same point in 1967 but only now is it openly debated. See also Smith, G. T. (1984) (editor) *A New NHS Act for 1996*? (papers prepared for a meeting 7–8 June 1984), Office of Health Economics, London.

CHAPTER 8

57. This was the quaint phrase used for a common event: married gentlewomen did not work then.
58. Miss Dorothy Atkins retired in 1973 to be succeeded by Miss Eileen Read until 1981 when Miss Lindsay Curtis took over. The Library Bulletin ceased publication on 1 January 1976: by then various other journals had taken on the same function, such as *Clinical Contents*.
59. See McMichael, J. (1952). 'Some problems of heart failure', *Acta Med. Scand.* Supplement 266, 701. Also Fowler, K. T. and Hyman, R. A. (1957) 'A mass spectrometer for rapid and continuous gas analysis'. *J. Physiol.* **137**, 33–35P.

CHAPTER 9

60 Sir Isaac Wolfson, knighted in 1962, with his brother Leonard established the Wolfson Foundation for advancement of health, education and youth activities. Also Chairman, Great Universal Stores, since 1946.
61. Sir Harold Himsworth was Professor of Medicine at University College Hospital 1939–1949 and Secretary of the Medical Research Council 1949–1968.
62. Earl King, see ref. 30, was a Canadian all his life and had considerable influence in Canada: he was therefore a very successful fund-raiser.
63. Lord Stamp had been Reader at the School 1937–1948 and Professor of Bacteriology 1948–1970. When he retired he was presented with a silver salver engraved with the outline of the Commonwealth Building, for which he had worked so hard.
64. Newman, see ref. 5.
65. Connie O'Driscoll personally interviewed every member of staff appointed and every new student who came: she had coffee evenings at her flat in Ladbroke Grove for overseas students to get to know each other and make them feel at home. She had a tinkling laugh and only seemed depressed when talking about the No. 7 bus service.
66. Basil Ward (1902–1976) had been Professor of Architecture at the Royal College of Art.
67. *The Hospital Plan for England and Wales* (1962), HMSO, London. See also Allen, D. E. (1979) *Hospital Planning*, Pitman, Tunbridge Wells (he was a Social Scientist who examined the decision-making process for the 1962 Plan and makes interesting reading).
68. It was never spelt out how these would be used.
69. Sir George Godber (1966) 'The Postgraduate Medical School: the future', *Postgrad. Med. J.*, **42**, 744–747. He was Chief Medical Officer to the Ministry of Health at the time.
70. *Royal Commission on Medical Education 1965–1968* (1968), HMSO, London. Lord A. R. Todd, who was the Chairman and Professor of Organic Chemistry University of Cambridge 1944–1971, became the first Chancellor of the University of Strathclyde, Glasgow, in 1978.

CHAPTER 10

71. Sir John Wolfenden, Vice-Chancellor of Reading University 1950–1963, was Chairman of the University Grants Committee 1963–1968.
72. Lewis, R. and Maude, A. (1952) *Professional People*, Phoenix House, London.

CHAPTER 11

73. Professor George Gask (1875–1951), knighted in 1919, was a member of the Governing Body of the School, a member of the Medical Research Council and Vice-president of the Royal College of Surgeons.

74. Lauwerys, J. A. (1950) 'Methods of education', *Br. Med. J.*, **iii**, 471–474.
75. When Vic Harrison retired in 1971 he became the first Professor of Pathology at the new University of Ife, Nigeria, and stayed for 3 years.
76. See McMichael's paper – ref. 20 – and Welbourn, R. B. (1966) 'The training and education of a surgeon', *Proc. R. Soc. Med.*, **59**, 934–6; also Longmire, W. P. on p. 936 with his reference to the 1910 Flexner Report on U.S.A. medical schools.
77. Pickering, G. (1974) in *The Way Ahead in Medical Education*, edited by MacLachlan (see below). Sir George Pickering was Master of Pembroke College at the time, having retired from the Regius Chair of Medicine at the Radcliffe Infirmary, Oxford.
78. Pickering, G. and MacLachlan, G. (1974) in the final chapter, 'The Summing Up', of the report of a 2-day seminar on postgraduate medical education (a re-run of a similar meeting held in 1961 to see what progress had been made by 1974: very little). *The Way Ahead* (1974), edited by G. MacLachlan for the Nuffield Provincial Hospitals Trust, Oxford Unviersity Press, London.
79. Lord Flowers, an eminent physicist, was rector of Imperial College of Science and Technology since 1973.

CHAPTER 12

80. Goodenough, see ref. 10.
81. Eric Bywaters became the first British Empire Rheumatism Council Professor of Rheumatology in 1957 and retired in 1975.
82. E. P. Sharpey-Schafer (1908–1963) became Professor of Medicine at St Thomas's Hospital in 1948.
83. Sheila Sherlock became Professor of Medicine at the Royal Free Hospital in 1959, having been at the School since 1942, and retired in 1983. Hepatitis was a scourge of the Army in North Africa, with an appreciable mortality and considerable morbidity, in the U.S.A. Army stationed in Northern Ireland (having been inoculated against yellow fever!) and in India where at one hospital all doctors becoming infected had to grow a moustache: by 1946 all had moustaches!
84. Pappworth, M. H. (1967) *Human Guineapigs: experimentation on man*, Routledge & Kegan Paul (and reprinted by Penguin, 1970).
85. Jim Dempster wrote the first British textbook on experimental surgery, and became Reader in Experimental Surgery.
86. Ralph Shackman had been assistant to Grey Turner, to become Reader in Surgery in 1955 and Professor of Urology in 1961. He retired in 1975 and died in 1981.
87. Denis Melrose became Professor of Surgical Science in 1969.
88. Alan Moncrieff (1901–1971) was Professor of Child Health 1934–1964 and knighted in 1964.
89. Peter Tizard was Professor of Paediatrics at the School 1964–1972, became the first Professor of Paediatrics at the University of Oxford in 1972, and was knighted 1982.
90. The British Heart Foundation in 1984 supported 15 Chairs of Cardiology in Britian.
91. There have only been four doctors as Ministers of Health since 1919: Christopher Addison, Walter Elliot, David Owen, Gerard Vaughan.

CHAPTER 13

92. Machiavelli had written 400 years earlier: 'Where the end is good, the means will always be justified.'
93. Machiavelli is supposed to have said that 'the innovator has for enemies all those who have done well under the old conditions'; the Hammersmith recognized that tradition reinforced complacency and had encouraged the questioning of traditional practices.
94. *Health Service Cost Statements*. N.W. Thames R.H.A. for year 31 March 1983.
95. Statistics supplied by the Records Office, Hammersmith Hospital.

96. The number of centenarians had increased too, from about 200 in 1954 to 2000 in 1984 (Clarke, C. C. (1984) 'Hybrids and hybridity', *J. R. Soc. Med.*, **77**, 821–829, according to the records from Buckingham Palace).

CHAPTER 14

97. E. R. Griffiths, Managing Director since 1977 of J. Sainsbury Ltd. A lawyer, responsible for *NHS Management Enquiry*, 6 October 1983.
98. Merrison, A. (1979) *Report of the Royal Commission on the National Health Service*, HMSO, London. Sir Alec Merrison was Vice-Chancellor of Bristol University 1969–1984. See also (1978) *Working of the National Health Service*, HMSO, London.
99. 'Evidence for submission to the Royal Commission on Medical Education', January 1966 from the British Postgraduate Medical Federation, and a separate submission from the School dated December 1965. The number of qualified doctors who enrolled in the various institutes of the Federation in 1963–1964 was U.K. 1206: overseas 2146.
100. Norman Morris has been Professor of Obstetrics and Gynaecology at Charing Cross Hospital since 1958, was Dean of the Faculty of Medicine in the University of London 1971–1976 and Vice-Chancellor 1976–1980. He was also at Hammersmith 1950–1952.
101. Professor L. P. Le Quesne, Professor of Surgery at the Middlesex Hospital since 1963, has been Deputy Vice-Chancellor and Dean of the Faculty of Medicine in the University of London since 1980.
102. The Pater formula is a university method for calculating the money needed for equipment for new buildings.
103. This was a thoughtful action because obtaining a crest of arms is a lengthy and expensive business.

CHAPTER 15

104. Lord Robbins, see ref. 51.
105. Sir Frederick Dainton, Chancellor of the University of Sheffield since 1978 and Chairman of Council R.P.M.S. since 1980.
106. H. H. Blandford, a member of the Governing Body of the British Postgraduate Medical Federation since 1969 and of the School since 1962, was Honorary Treasurer from 1964.
107. Sir Frank Hartley, Dean of the School of Pharmacy 1962–1976, was Vice-Chancellor of the University 1976–1978.
108. R. B. Welbourn, Professor of Surgical Endocrinology since 1979, was Director of the Department of Surgery 1963–1979 and a Member of Council 1971–1975.
109. Robert Steiner, Professor of Diagnostic Radiology since 1961, was a previous Chairman of the Academic Board.
110. Nick Wright was Professor of Histopathology at the School.

CHAPTER 16

111. Peter Drucker, Professor of Management at New York University's Graduate School of Business, was a prolific writer on organization, administration and management.
112. Christopher Hogg, Chairman of Courtaulds Ltd since 1980.
113. Lord Arnold Weinstock, Managing Director since 1963 of General Electric Ltd.
114. Kearns, W. (1984) 'Mothers and children: research priorities', *J. R. Soc. Med.*, **77**, 356–7.
115. A copy of the report is filed in the Wellcome Library of the R.P.M.S.
116. Lord Rayner, who became Chairman of Marks and Spencer plc in 1984, instituted cost-cutting scrutinies for the Secretary of State for Social Services.
117. Said by Ian MacGregor, Chairman of the National Coal Board, in a radio interview in 1984.

Appendix I

List of Floors in the Commonwealth Building

10th Floor:	The Sieff Surgical Clinical Laboratories
9th Floor:	The Max Rayne Cardiovascular Laboratories and The Wellcome Laboratories of Clinical Pharmacology
8th Floor:	The Blandford Laboratories of Bacteriology
7th Floor:	The Wellcome Laboratories of Virology, of Chemical Microbiology and of Cell Biology
6th Floor:	The Canada Laboratories of Chemical Pathology
5th Floor:	Histochemistry, Biophysics and Steroid Biochemistry Laboratories
4th Floor:	Haematology Laboratories including the Wellcome Laboratories of Tropical Haematology
3rd Floor:	The Commonwealth Teaching Laboratories and the South African Museum
2nd Floor:	Administration and Medical Photography
1st Floor:	The Wellcome Library
Ground Floor:	Entrance Hall, Medical Illustration and Library Stack Room
Lower Ground Floor:	Medical Physics Laboratories and Medical School Stores
Basement:	Small animals

Appendix II

Staff and Departments

CLINICAL STAFF IN 1940/1941

Administration

Dean, Colonel Proctor; Sub-dean, Dr C. E. Newman; Assistant Secretary, Miss C. O'Driscoll; Librarian, Miss D. F. Atkins (Mr Lloyd had joined the Army).
Total = 4.

Department of Medicine

Director, Professor F. R. Fraser; Reader, Dr J. McMichael; Senior Assistant (L.C.C.), Dr T. St. C. Norris; First Assistants, Dr J. G. Scadding, Dr P. H. Wood, Dr E. P. Sharpey-Schafer, Dr N. S. Allcock; Part-time Assistant, Dr E. G. L. Bywaters; Dermatologist, Dr R. T. Brain; Psychologist, Dr A. J. Lewis; Neurologist, Dr J. P. Martin; Paediatrician, Dr R. Lightwood.
Total = 12

Department of Surgery

Director, Professor Grey Turner; Reader, Mr A. K. Henry; Senior Assistant (L.C.C.) Mr G. C. Dorling; First Assistants, Mr Ruscoe Clarke, Mr D. M. Douglas, Mr R. H. Franklin; visiting surgeon (Thyroid cases), Sir Thomas Dunhill; Assistant (Throat, Nose and Ear), Mr J. L. Griffiths; Assistant (Neuro-Surgery), Mr G. C. Knight; Ophthalmic Surgeon, Mr P. M. Moffatt; Honorary Consultant for Venereal Diseases, Colonel L. W. Harrison; Anaesthetist, Dr H. Woodfield Davies; Resident Anaesthetist, Dr Dorothy Spence-Sales.
Total = 13.

Department of Obstetrics and Gynaecology

Director, Professor James Young; Reader, Dr R. J. Kellar; Senior Assistant (L.C.C.), Dr A. B. Field; First Assistant, Dr M. Kenny; Visiting Obstetrician and Gynaecologist, Mr. V. B. Green-Armytage; Anaesthetist, Dr Dorothy Spence-Sales.
Total = 6

Department of Pathology

Director, Professor J. Henry Dible; Reader (Pathological Chemisry), Dr E. J. King; Reader (Morbid Anatomy), vacant – Dr J. Gray had resigned due to ill-health in 1939; Reader (Bacteriology), Lord Stamp; Senior Assistant (Clinical Pathology), Dr Janet Vaughan; Senior Assistant (Morbid Anatomy), Dr T. H. Belt; Assistant (Pathological Chemistry), Dr D. Beall; Assistant (Morbid Anatomy), Dr A. I. Ross and Dr J. W. Clegg; Assistant (Bacteriology), Dr Mary Barber and Dr D. M. Stone.
Total = 10

Department of Radiology (entirely L.C.C. appointed)

Director, Dr J. Duncan White; Assistant, Dr E. J. E. Topham; Physicist, Dr L. H. S. Clark.
Total = 3

Medical Superintendent of Hammersmith Hospital

Sir Thomas Carey Evans.

GRAND TOTAL = 49

CLINICAL STAFF IN 1960/1961

Administration

Dean, Dr Charles Newman; Secretary, Constance O'Driscoll; Accountant, Mr G. A. Barnes; Librarian, Dorothy F. Atkins; Consulting Statistician, Mr N. W. Please.
Total = 5

Department of Medicine

Director, Professor J. McMichael; Professor of Endocrinology and Assistant Director, Professor T. Russell Fraser; Empire Rheumatism Council Professor of Rheumatology, E. G. L. Bywaters; Reader in Metabolic Diseases, Dr C. L. Cope; Senior Lecturers, Dr C. M. Fletcher and Dr J. F. Goodwin; Lecturers, Dr C. C. Booth, Dr A. S. Dixon, Dr A. Hollman, Dr M. Milne, Dr J. P. D. Mounsey, Dr C. Pallis, Dr O. M. Wrong; Honorary Assistant Lecturers, Dr C. Dollery and Dr I. Gabe.

All the above were full-time. Part-time staff were:
Senior Lecturer, Dr J. Shillingford; Lecturers, Dr P. Hugh-Jones and Dr P. Strandling (Tuberculosis).
Sessional staff were:
Senior Lecturer (chest diseases), Dr J. G. Scadding; Lecturers, Dr B. Ackner (Psychological Medicine), Dr I. C. Gilliland (Geriatrics), Dr S. C. Gold (Dermatology).
Total = 22

Department of Surgery

Director, Professor Ian Aird; Professor of Urology, R. Shackman; Readers, W. J. Dempster (Experimental Surgery) and D. G. Melrose (Clinical Rheology); Lecturers, H. H. Bentall (Cardiac Surgery), W. H. Stephenson (Orthopaedics), J. S. Calnan (Experimental Plastic Surgery), Assistant Lecturer (Cardiac Pathology), Dr Monica Bishop.
All the above were full-time. Part-time staff were:
Senior Lecturer, Mr W. P. Cleland (Thoracic Surgery), Mr R. H. Franklin, Mr C. Gray (Orthopaedics), Mr I. Griffiths (Otolaryngology), Mr G. C. Knight (Neurosurgery), Mr P. M. G. Moffatt (Opthalmology), Mr J. N. Barron (Plastic Surgery); Lecturers, Mr H. D. Johnson (General Surgery), Mr Peter Martin (Vascular Surgery), Mr A. K. Monro (General Surgery), Mr Selwyn Taylor (General Surgery).
Total = 20

Anaesthesia

Lecturers, Dr J. P. Payne and M. K. Sykes, both whole-time.
Visiting consultants were: Senior Lecturer, Dr H. Woodfield-Davies; Lecturers, Dr A. J. W. Beard, Dr Dorothy Spence-Sales, Dr F. G. Wood-Smith, Dr Elizabeth Lloyd-Jones and Dr J. F. Nunn.
Total = 8

Department of Pathology

Chairman: Professor E. J. King.
Section of Bacteriology: Professor, Lord Stamp; Reader, Dr Mary Barber; Senior Lecturers, Dr W. Hayes and Dr D. A. Mitchison; Lecturer, Dr Naomi Datta; Assistant Lecturer, Dr A. C. Dutton.
Section of Biophysics: Senior Lecturer, D. K. Hill, Dr E. H. Belcher; Honorary Lecturers in Medical Physics, J. F. Fowler and Dr J. R. Mallard; Leverhulme Lecturer in Medical Engineering (electronics), Mr. E. Pallett.
Section of Chemical Pathology: Professor E. J. King; Reader, Dr I. D. P. Wootton; Honorary Senior Lecturers, Dr G. E. Dalgleish and Dr G. Popjak; Lecturer, Dr I. MacIntyre; Assistant Lecturers, Dr D. W. Moss and Dr Ruth Haslam; Honorary Assistant Lecturer, Dr R. W. Dutton.
Section of Haematology: Professor J. V. Dacie; Senior Lecturers, Dr J. C. White and Dr D. L. Mollin; Lecturer, Dr S. M. Lewis; Honorary Lecturer (part-time), Dr D. Galton; Honorary Assistant Lecturer, Dr Leon Szur.
Section of Morbid Anatomy: Professor C. V. Harrison; Reader, vacant; Reader in Histochemistry, Dr A. G. E. Pearse; Lecturer, Dr B. E. Heard; Assistant Lecturer, Dr J. G. Azzopardi.
Total = 31

Department of Diagnostic Radiology

Director, Professor R. E. Steiner; Senior Lecturer, Dr J. W. Laws; Assistant Lecturer, Dr F. H. Doyle.
Total = 3

Department of Radiotheraphy

Director and Senior Lecturer, Dr Constance A. P. Wood; Lecturers, Dr R. Morrison, Dr Lilian H. Walter and Dr A. W. Goolden.
Total = 4

Medical Superintendent of Hammersmith Hospital

Dr C. E. Roberts (who succeeded Dr Wimbush and Sir Carey Evans, in 1958).

Chest Clinic

Dr P. Stradling.
Total = 2

GRAND TOTAL 95

CLINICAL STAFF IN 1980/1981

Administration

Dean, Dr Malcolm Godfrey; Vice-Deans, Professor D. W. Moss and Dr R. E. Eban (Ealing Hospital); Secretary, Dr J. R. Welsman; Deputy Secretary, Mr A. Ingle; Senior Assistant Secretary, Mr N. Gershon; Accommodations Officer, Mr G. H. Vellacott (previous School Secretary 1965–1977); Financial Secretary, Mr W. W. Windsor; Accountants, Mr J. M. Digby, Mr E. J. H. Lloyd, Mr D. A. W. Harris; Librarian, Miss E. M. Read; Assistant Librarian, Miss A. R. L. Mapplebeck.
Total = 13

Department of Medicine

Director, Professor D. K. Peters; Professor of Clinical Cardiology, J. F. Goodwin; Sir John McMichael Professor of Cardiovascular Medicine, A. Maseri; Professor of Geriatric Medicine, H. M. Hodkinson; Reader in Medicine, Dr S. R. Bloom; Reader in Clinical Endocrinology, Dr G. F. Joplin; Reader in Neurology, Dr C. Pallis; Reader in Immunology, Dr M. B. Pepys; Senior Lecturers, Dr V. S. Chadwick (Gastroenterology), Dr H. J. F. Hodgson (Gastroenterology), Dr G. R. V. Hughes (Rheumatology), Dr J. M. B. Hughes (Respiratory Medicine), Dr C. M. Lockwood (Renal Medicine), Dr J. G. P. Sisson (Medicine); Lecturer, Dr S. Chierchia

(Cardiology); Honorary Senior Lecturers, Dr M. G. Impallomeni (Geriatric Medicine), Dr Eva M. Kohner (Medical Ophthalmology), Dr N. J. Legg (Neurology), Dr Celia M. Oakley (Clinical Cardiology), Dr G. W. Poole (Respiratory Diseases), Dr N. B. Pride (Respiratory Diseases), Dr A. J. Rees (Renal Medicine); Honorary Lecturer, Dr Katherine A. Hallidie-Smith (Paediatric Cardiology), Dr H. Mashiter (Endocrinology), Dr A. P. Selwyn (Cardiovascular Medicine).
The above were all full-time. The sessional staff were:
Senior Lecturers, Dr L. A. Hersov (Psychological Medicine), Dr H. R. Vickers (Dermatology); Honorary Senior Lecturers, Dr K. P. Fink (Psychological Medicine), Dr I. C. Lodge-Patch (Psychological Medicine), Dr P. I. Reed and Dr A. Jadresic (Endocrinology), Dr J. Reeve (Nuclear Medicine), Dr L. H. Sevitt (Renal Medicine), Dr G. Woolfson (Psychological Medicine); Honorary Senior Research Fellows, Dr A. J. Barnes (Endocrinology), Dr R. Blackwood (Cardiology), Dr J. Cassar (Endocrinology).

Ealing Hospital

Honorary Senior Lecturers: Dr Charlotte Feldman (Rheumatology), Dr D. M. Krikler (Cardiovascular Disease), Dr H. B. McMichael (Gastroenterology) and Dr H. Rudolf (Respiratory Diseases).
Total, excluding Ealing = 37.

Department of Surgery

Director, Professor L. H. Blumgart; Professor of Cardiac Surgery, H. H. Bentall; Professor of Plastic and Reconstructive Surgery, J. S. Calnan; Professor of Surgical Science, D. G. Melrose; Professor of Experimental Pathology, H. K. Weinbren; Professor of Surgical Endocrinology, R. B. Welbourn; Senior Lecturers, J. Spencer (General Surgery), C. B. Wood (General Surgery), D. Mee (Urology); Honorary Senior Lecturers, J. Schrager (General Surgery), M. P. Singh (Paediatric Surgery), G. Williams (Urology/Renal); Lecturers, I. S. Benjamin (General Surgery), R. T. Mathie (Surgical Physiology).
All the above were full-time. The sessional staff were:
Professor of Neurosurgery (at the Institute of Neurology), L. Symon; Senior Lecturers, J. H. Baron (Gastroenterology), R. Ghanadian, C. W. Jamieson (Vascular), R. N. Sapsford (Cardiothoracic); Honorary Senior Lecturers, P. J. Bourdillon (Clinical Physiology), J. P. S. England (Orthopaedics), P. K. Leaver (Ophthalmology) and J. Pflug (Venous and Lymphatic).

Ealing Hospital

Honorary Senior Lecturers: A. E. Carter (General Surgery), M. J. Evans (Orthopaedics), J. A. Lynn (General Surgery), G. Jantet (Vascular).
Total, excluding Ealing = 24.

Department of Anaesthetics

Director, Professor J. G. Robson; Reader, J. G. Whitwam; Senior Lecturers, G. M. Hall and M. Morgan; Honorary Lecturers, L. Loh, Jean Lumley and C. D. Richards.
All the above were full-time. The sessional staff were:
Honorary Senior Lecturer, R. D. Jack.

Ealing Hospital

Senior Lecturer, Ruth Owen.
Total, excluding Ealing = 7.

Department of Clinical Pharmacology

Director, Professor C. T. Dollery; Professor of Biochemical Pharmacology, D. S. Davies; Senior Lecturers in Clinical Pharmacology, P. J. Lewis and C. J. Bulpitt (Honorary); Lecturers, I. A. Blair (Analytical Chemistry), A. R. Boobis (Biochemical Pharmacology), M. J. Brown; Honorary Lecturer, P. I. Harris.
Total = 8

Division of Pathology

Chairman, Professor D. A. Mitchison.

Department of Bacteriology

Director, Professor D. A. Mitchison; Professor of Microbiological Genetics, Naomi Datta; Reader in Clinical Bacteriology, J. H. Darrell; Lecturer, R. W. Hedges; Honorary Senior Lecturer, W. G. Henderson; Honorary Lecturers, Jean M. E. Dickinson and D. B. Lowne.

Department of Chemical Pathology

Director, Professor I. D. P. Wootton; Professor of Endocrine Chemistry, I. MacIntyre; Professor of Clinical Enzymology, D. W. Moss; Reader, Dr K. Fotherby; Senior Lecturers, Dr Heather G. M. Freeman and Dr M. Szelke.

Department of Haematology

Director, Professor L. Luzatto; Reader, Dr S. M. Lewis; Senior Lecturer, Dr E. C. Gordon-Smith; Honorary Senior Lecturer, Dr U. M. Hegde; Professor of Haematological Oncology (MRC Leukaemia Unit) D. A. G. Calton; Honorary Senior Lecturers, Dr D. Catovsky and Dr J. M. Goldman.

Department of Histopathology

Director, Professor N. A. Wright; Professor of Oncology, J. C. Azzopardi; Professor of Histochemistry, A. G. E. Pearse; Professor of Tissue Pathology, D. J. Evans; Senior Lecturers, Dr P. D. Lewis (Neuropathology), Dr Elizabeth E. Pearse (Cytology), Dr Julia M. Polak (Histochemistry); Lecturer in Experimental Pathology, Dr M. R. Alison; Honorary Senior Lecturers, Dr P. D. Byers, Dr I. A. Lampert and Dr Julia Denekamp.

Department of Immunology

Director, Professor J. H. Humphrey; Professor of Tissue Immunology, Dr J. R. Batchelor; Senior Lecturers, Dr C. J. F. Spry and Dr B. D. Williams.

Department of Virology

Director, Professor A. P. Waterson; Senior Lecturers, Dr Gundrum Agnarsdottir and Dr K. Apostolov.
Total = 38

Department of Medical Physics

Director, Professor J. S. Orr; Professor of Biophysics, Dr D. K. Hill; Reader, Dr E. W. Emery; Honorary Senior Lecturers, Dr G. R. Ball (Medical Engineering), Dr R. E. Trotman, Dr N. Veall (Radioisotopes); Lecturer, J. E. Pallett (Medical Engineering and Electronics); Honorary Lecturer, Dr M. J. Myers; Honorary Senior Research Fellow, Dr P. Merton.
Total = 9

Department of Diagnostic Radiology

Director, Professor R. E. Steiner; Professor of Radiological Sciences, F. H. Doyle; Senior Lecturer, N. B. Bowley; Honorary Senior Lecturers, D. J. Allison, R. E. Eban, J. P. Lavender and B. E. Nathan.
Total = 7

Department of Paediatrics and Neonatal Medicine

Director, Professor V. Dubowitz; Readers, Pamela A. Davies (Paediatrics), J. S. Wigglesworth (Paediatric Pathology); Senior Lecturer, M. Silverman; Honorary Senior Lecturer, A. G. L. Whitelaw; Senior Biochemist, Elizabeth A. Hughes.
Total = 6

Department of Obstetrics and Gynaecology

Director, Professor M. G. Elder; Professor of Obstetric Therapeutics, D. F. Hawkins; Reader, W. G. MacGregor; Senior Lecturer, R. M. L. Winston; Lecturers, W. Gillett and L. Myatt (Biochemistry).
All the above were full-time. Sessional staff were:
Senior Lecturers, J. L. Fluker (Venerology), L. Goldie (Medical Psychotherapy), J. C. O'Sullivan (Oncology); Honorary Senior Lecturers in Research, Lilly H. Zondek and T. Zondek; Honorary Lecturer, Anne V. Tothill.
Total = 12

Department of Radiotheraphy (Hammersmith Hospital)

Director and Honorary Senior Lecturer, K. E. Halnan; Honorary Senior Lecturers, Mary Catterall, A. W. G. Goolden, Hannah E. Lambert and C. G. McKenzie.
Total = 5

Cyclotron Unit (Medical Research Council)

Director and Honorary Lecturer in Physics, D. D. Vonberg; Honorary Lecturers, D. K. Bewley (Medical Physics), S. B. Field (Medical Physics) Shirley Hornsey (Radiopathology), C. J. Parnell (Medical Physics) and D. J. Silvester (Radiochemistry).
Total = 6

Lipid Metabolism (Medical Research Council)

Director and Honorary Senior Lecturer, N. B. Myant (Chemical Pathology); Honorary Senior Lecturer, G. R. Thompson (Medicine).
Total = 2

General Practitioner Educational Activities

Clinical Tutor, Pamela A. Davies; Senior Tutor in General Practice, S. J. Carne.
Total = 2

Animal Science

Senior Lecturer, P. N. O'Donoghue.
Total = 1

Computing Science

Senior Lecturer, P. J. Vitek.
Total = 1

GRAND TOTAL = 168.

Index

The names of members of staff in post in 1940, 1960, and 1980 are contained in Appendix II. They are not included here unless directly connected with events recorded in the text.

GPSR Compliance

The European Union's (EU) General Product Safety Regulation (GPSR) is a set of rules that requires consumer products to be safe and our obligations to ensure this.

If you have any concerns about our products, you can contact us on ProductSafety@springernature.com

In case Publisher is established outside the EU, the EU authorized representative is:

Springer Nature Customer Service Center GmbH
Europaplatz 3
69115 Heidelberg, Germany

Batch number: 10607212

Printed by Printforce, the Netherlands